Children/Youth Physical Fitness Program Management System

A management system to aid school administrators, physical education teachers, and professional preparation instructors in developing and directing a physical fitness program.

A project of the City and County Directors Council ARAPCS/AAHPERD

by

Lou Mozzini, formerly San Diego County Office of Education
Bob Pestolesi, University of Southern California
Bob Pangrazi, Arizona State University (Principal reviewer)

ii

About the Alliance

The American Alliance is an educational organization, structured for the purposes of supporting, encouraging, and providing assistance to member groups and their personnel throughout the nation as they seek to initiate, develop, and conduct programs in health, leisure, and movement-related activities for the enrichment of human life.

Alliance objectives include:

1. Professional growth and development—to support, encourage, and provide guidance in the development and conduct of programs in health, leisure, and movement-related activities which are based on the needs, interests, and inherent capacities of the individual in today's society.

2. Communication—to facilitate public and professional understanding and appreciation of the importance and value of health, leisure, and movement-related activities as they contribute toward human well-being.

3. Research—to encourage and facilitate research which will enrich the depth and scope of health, leisure, and movement-related activities; and to disseminate the findings to the profession and other interested and concerned publics.

4. Standards and guidelines—to further the continuous development and evaluation of standards within the profession for personnel and programs in health, leisure, and movement-related activities.

5. Public affairs—to coordinate and administer a planned program of professional, public, and governmental relations that will improve education in areas of health, leisure, and movement-related activities.

6. To conduct such other activities as shall be approved by the Board of Governors and the Alliance Assembly, provided that the Alliance shall not engage in any activity which would be inconsistent with the status of an educational and charitable organization as defined in Section 501(c) (3) of the Internal Revenue Code of 1954 or any successor provision thereto, and none of the said purposes shall at any time be deemed or construed to be purposes other than the public benefit purposes and objectives consistent with such educational and charitable status.   *Bylaws, Article III*

The *Children/Youth Physical Fitness Program Management System* was developed as a project of the City and County Directors Council of the Association for Research, Administration, Professional Councils, and Societies (ARAPCS). Lou Mozzini, then council chairperson and coordinator of health and physical education with the San Diego Office of Education, developed the management system and the major portion of the program content. Bob Pestolesi, University of Southern California, provided valuable assistance and direction in both format and content, and was responsible for developing the management planning steps. Bob Pangrazi, Arizona State University, acted as the principal reviewer. His valuable critique of each management stage has added credibility to the publication as a viable tool for both elementary and secondary school personnel and college and university faculty in administering children and youth physical fitness programs.

About the Authors

Introduction

Today there are more boys and girls participating in sports than at any other time in the history of our nation. The adults of our country are daily subscribing to health spas, fitness centers, and industrial sports and fitness programs. They have discovered that engaging in physical activity can make you look and feel better, and, if done properly, can be an exciting, enjoyable, and worthwhile experience.

Evidence continues to show a positive relationship between physical activity and health and wellness. Recent studies support the fact that those individuals who are physically fit reduce the risk of coronary heart disease, do better in academic learning, are less susceptible to stress, have greater independence, greater control of aggression, and are less obese.

Knowing this, why then do we find our school age children less fit today than their counterparts in the 1960's? The answer to this question may be related to a general sedentary lifestyle, coupled with a decrease in professional fitness educators in the schools, the lack of a systematic approach to teaching physical fitness to children, a lack of legal requirements to report fitness scores at the district and state levels, and minimal supervision of the programs by principals, physical education directors, and district supervisors.

Motor skill improvement and physical fitness development are equally important ingredients of any comprehensive school physical education program. Physical fitness should be only a part of the school's physical education curriculum and should not be seen as the total physical education program. Physical fitness is an important component of a well-rounded physical education program and must be designed to meet the individual and group needs of all school age children. The system presented in this publication is designed to take you, the physical fitness program manager, through the process of justification, evaluation, development, supervision, and promotion of a sound physical fitness program.

A commitment to the achievement of a comprehensive physical fitness curriculum will help to ensure that our children will grow into fully functioning, healthy adults.

How to Use the System

The *Children/Youth Physical Fitness Program Management System* is designed to be used in various ways depending on the needs of program administrators. There are seven management stages for administrators to work through in managing a children/youth physical fitness program. Management stage 1.0 includes a program assessment instrument to guide the administrator in determining program needs and help identify the system management stages that will assist in managing a physical fitness program. If some management stages have been achieved, administrators should focus on the priority areas identified in the program assessment instrument.

Each management stage includes one or more management objectives simply stated to provide direction to the administrator in completing the management stage. Some management objectives will specify a product to be developed, while others identify functions to be performed. It is not necessary to achieve each management objective sequentially, but rather, focus on identified nonfunctioning program areas.

Management planning steps suggest various actions the administrator should take to accomplish the management objective. Sample activities, and sometimes sample products are suggested for each management planning step. These samples are suggestions only; administrators should examine them to determine the feasibility of each to their own program.

Reference material to support products or functions are listed for each management objective. References listed are limited and are provided as suggestions only.

Management Stages

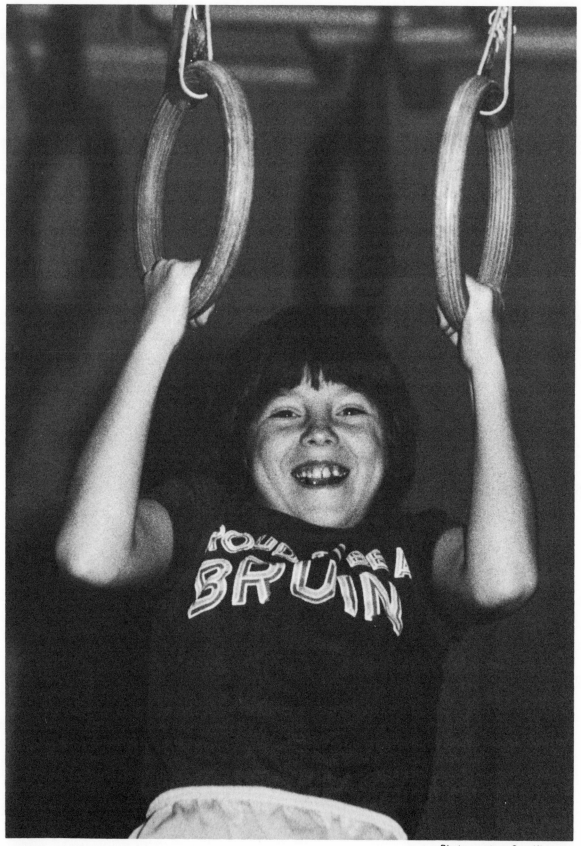

Photo courtesy Sue Klemens.

1.0

PROGRAM ASSESSMENT

Includes an assessment instrument to determine program needs and set priorities by referring administrators to various management objectives for program development.

Management Objective

Management Objective 1.1

Assess the Children/Youth Physical Fitness Program in Your School or District

Management Planning Steps:

Step One   Conduct an assessment to determine the operational level of the existing physical fitness program.

Step Two   Determine needs and set priorities for program development or improvement.

Sample Assessment Procedures

Program Assessment

The assessment instrument is designed to assist the program administrator in determining the operational level of the existing physical fitness program. The effects of school physical fitness programs are long lasting. For these effects to be beneficial, physical fitness programs must be sound. To make them sound, program administrators should operate under a planned sequential management system.

The assessment instrument is divided into seven management stages which are essential to successful program administration. Each management stage includes from one to seven related management objectives which provide direction to the program administrator toward the achievement of each management stage. The assessment design will permit users to match the functioning level of their existing program with the recommended program management system objectives.

Setting Program Priorities

The program management system has been presented sequentially by development stages. Priorities for program development are determined by the order of nonfunctioning management objectives identified by the assessment instrument.

Program Assessment Instrument

Management Stage[1]	Operational Level		Management Objective Reference
	Functioning	Nonfunctioning	
2.0 PROGRAM COMMITMENT			
• A plan is developed to solicit a regular sustained commitment for the physical fitness program			2.1
3.0 PROGRAM PLANNING			
• A physical fitness program as part of the total physical education curriculum is developed			3.0

[1] There are seven Management Stages. Management Stage 1.0, Program Assessment, describes the program assessment process.

Management Stage	Operational Level		Management Objective Reference
	Functioning	Nonfunctioning	
4.0 PROGRAM IMPLEMENTATION— ADMINISTRATIVE FUNCTIONS			
• Legal statutes which govern the physical fitness program are identified			4.1
• A budget is developed and approved which grants sufficient funds for the physical fitness program			4.2
• A criteria is developed for staff qualifications which will facilitate student accomplishment of the program objectives			4.3
• Appropriate facilities and equipment are available for the physical fitness program			4.4
• Appropriate instructional materials, audiovisual aids, and program supplies are provided for the physical fitness program			4.5
5.0 PROGRAM IMPLEMENTATION— INSTRUCTIONAL FUNCTIONS			
• A physical fitness test battery which assesses the level of all students is utilized			5.1
• A computer is utilized for processing test information, facilitating instruction, and storing data			5.2
• Professional support is provided to staff on administration and test results utilization			5.3
• Professional support is provided to staff on the principles of exercise and instructional approaches			5.4
• Professional support is provided to staff on the various aspects which cause physical fitness instruction to be safe and beneficial			5.5
• Professional support is provided to staff on conducting developmental physical fitness programs specific to individual student needs			5.6
• A program is developed which will provide an incentive for students, staff, and school to continually seek higher goals			5.7
6.0 PUBLIC RELATIONS			
• A public relations program is conducted regularly for the purpose of creating awareness of the value of children/youth physical fitness programs			6.1
7.0 PROGRAM SUPERVISION AND EVALUATION			
• A procedure to supervise and evaluate operation of the children/youth physical fitness program management system is operational			7.1

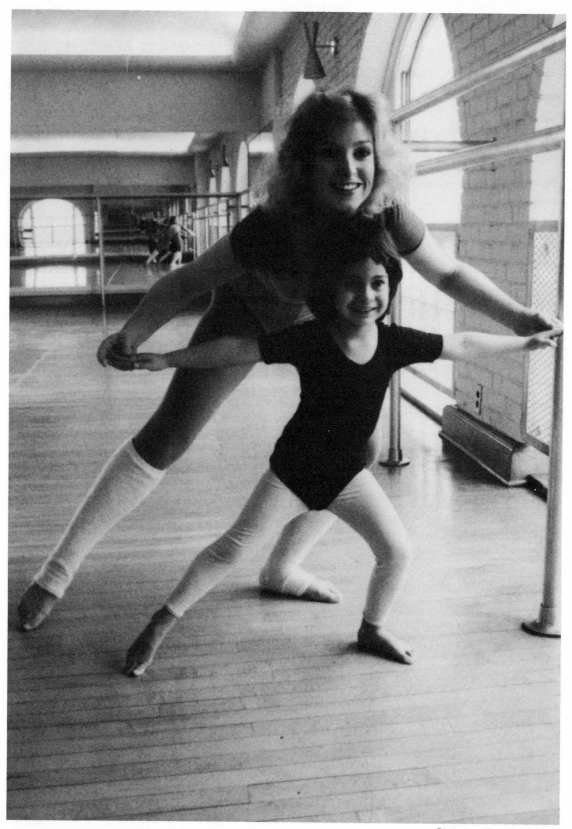

Photo courtesy Karen Hall.

2.0

PROGRAM COMMITMENT

Includes support materials and a strategy to solicit regular sustained commitment for a comprehensive children/youth physical fitness program.

**Management
Objective**

Management Objective 2.1

> ## Enlist Support and Commitment for a Children/Youth Physical Fitness Program
>
> ### Management Planning Steps:
>
> Step One — Compile a packet of support materials justifying the needs and purposes for a physical fitness program.
>
> Step Two — Enlist commitment from the instructional staff to conduct a strong physical fitness program at all levels.
>
> Step Three — Obtain support from the local governing board, school administration, and community for a continued physical fitness program.

Sample Plan to Enlist Committment and Support

Support Materials Packet

Program administrators need to compile a packet of written and audio-visual materials justifying the value of physical fitness and its importance as part of a comprehensive physical education program. The written materials should include:

- Recent and significant research
- Basic beliefs and recommendations
- Indicators for quality elementary school programs
- Indicators for quality secondary school programs

The audiovisual portion of the packet should include a visual display and audio presentation depicting the significance, value, and justification of a strong school fitness curriculum. If a successful local school program is in operation, program administration should develop an audiovisual presentation in support of physical fitness.

Recent and significant research

Coronary heart disease is responsible for 55% of the deaths in the western world. Risk factors associated with the onset of the disease in adults are now identifiable in children (Wilmore and McNamara, 1974; Lauer et al., 1975; and Gilliam et al., 1977). Physical activity of an aerobic nature (20 minutes continuous, at one's target heart rate, three times per week) has been found to have a positive effect on three of these risk factors: 1) serum blood lipid levels, 2) obesity, and 3) physical inactivity.

Blood Lipids
Two recent studies (Gilliam and Burke, 1978; and Thorland and Gilliam, 1981) have indicated that involvement in intense physical activity may be associated with the maintenance of desirable lipid levels in children. Seefeldt (Grant Proposal, 1982) states that "the study by Gilliam and Burke (1978) further indicated the importance of continued vigorous activity in that the desirable serum lipid levels regressed to pretraining levels after discontinuation of the physical activity program."

Obesity
Fat cell multiplication occurs at the fastest rate during two periods in a person's life: 1) the third trimester of pregnancy through the first year, and 2) between the ages of nine to thirteen years of age. Four studies (Johnson, et al., 1964; Wilmore and McNamara, 1974; Lauer et al., 1975; and Gilliam, et al., 1977) have identified obesity as a problem among preadolescents. Three additional studies have indicated that inactivity, and not diet, may be the major cause of obesity (Corbin and Pletcher, 1968; Bullen, et al., 1975; and Mayer, 1974).

Physical inactivity
Physical inactivity is the major cause of obesity. Three studies have suggested that children do *not* engage in a high enough level of activity (target heart rate—85% of maximum heart rate) for an adequate amount of time (20 minutes) to improve their cardiovascular fitness (Hovell, et al., 1978; Gilliam, et al., 1981; and Gilliam et al., 1982). Gilliam et al., (1982) also found that the activity levels of the children were significantly higher following an eight week exercise program.

Physical fitness levels are inadequate among youth. Evidence from many different viewpoints supports the need to improve the level of physical performance. Three national studies indicate that fitness levels have not increased over the last two decades due to a lack of emphasis on physical fitness by physical educators.

Some programs have succeeded in enhancing youth fitness. In particular, the Positively Fit program, the La Sierra program, and the Cincinnati Academy of Physical Education are examples of school programs which have received national recognition for their ability to enhance physical fitness among youth. Fitness performance can be improved and programs are available for doing so. If fitness is not promoted in physical education programs, it could lead youngsters to believe that fitness is not important for a healthy, well-balanced lifestyle.

More than ever before, fitness is on center stage. If professionals cannot sell the importance of fitness to the public today, they may never be able to do so. Physical educators must take advantage of the constant media barrage of wellness information and methods.

Coaches have access to a great deal of information on how to keep a larger number of students involved in sport. Yet because more than 80 percent of students drop out of interscholastic sports, other opportunities need to be made available to them. Private agencies are developing programs that appeal to youth. Training programs for youth coaches need to be developed and required.

Future lifetime sports programs must develop functional fitness for recreational and leisure time participation. In a sense, youngsters have been expected to participate in sports programs without having developed adequate physical fitness and motor skills to do so.

Women are immensely interested in personal fitness. School fitness programs must consider the interests and needs of both sexes and modify programs accordingly. Intramural programs need to continue to broaden the number of activities offered.

Basic beliefs and recommendations

A renewed concern for creative fitness programs that turn high school students on instead of off needs to be developed. Fitness programs, available for children and for adults, have forgotten students in grades 7-12.

Pangrazi (1984) discusses the need for programs which focus on fitness that promotes health. Programs of physical training or the single-minded "daily dozen and run a mile approach" do not serve students for a lifetime. Students must understand why fitness is important, how to evaluate their personal fitness, and what to prescribe for personal exercise programs.

Hayes (1984) describes some of the requirements for every school's physical fitness program. Hayes indicates that all school children in grades kindergarten through twelve should be required to participate in daily programs of physical education which emphasize the development of physical fitness and skills for growth and development, and encourage a lifetime of vigor and health. Every pupil should be tested in physical fitness at least twice a year, and should have an understanding of the basic principles of exercise science and how to apply them.

Every pupil should have posture checks, body composition assessments, and routine health screenings with appropriate follow-up. Underdeveloped pupils should be given appropriate remedial attention, and disabled students should be identified and provided with appropriate programs.

American children and adolescents are not developing the exercise and fitness skills that could help maintain their good health as adults, and as many as half may not be getting enough exercise to develop healthy cardiorespiratory systems, according to a two-year nationwide study released by Department of Health and Human Services Secretary Margaret M. Heckler (1984). The study, funded by the U.S. Public Health Service Office of Disease Prevention and Health Promotion, surveyed 8,800 students across the nation in grades five through 12. The survey examined fitness and exercise habits. In addition, rigorous physical tests were administered which, for the first time in such a study, were designed to show overall health and fitness rather than athletic ability or agility.

Heckler states that "This study should serve as a warning. It shows that America's school children are not achieving the lifetime fitness skills required to promote good health ... but it can also serve us as a blueprint for achieving the exercise and fitness goals we seek for today's children and the generations to come."

Indicators of quality preschool and elementary school programs

Preschool level

The term physical fitness is not commonly associated with educational programs for preschool children. There are several reasons for this apparent omission: first, most preschool curricula emphasize the development of fine motor, social, and cognitive skills, to the neglect of gross motor activities and fitness. Some incidental large motor development may take place in these settings, but this is primarily as a consequence of play. Seldom do preschool children have access to a defined program of gross motor skills, wherein the progressions of patterns that lead to proficiency in our games, sports, and dances are taught in a systematic manner. Second, the components of physical fitness, as they are identified in most factor analytic studies on older individuals, may be of secondary importance in early childhood. For young children, the commonly defined fitness components of endurance, flexibility, and strength are by-products of learning the fundamental motor skills essential for locomotion and play.

Elementary level
In physical education programs for elementary school children, it is time to reexamine what we are trying to accomplish and whether our objectives are in concert with those who support public education.

The selection of objectives for elementary school physical education programs is a straightforward matter if educators apply criteria that address the concerns of expectations, feasibility, and outcome. The objectives must be unique to physical activity programs; they must address the notion of order, sequence, and developmental level in the behaviors that are to be changed; and they must define the changes in skills, knowledge, and attitudes that will result from participation in the program.

Seefeldt (1984) indicates that changing children's activity patterns requires a four-step process. First, we must communicate to parents and administrators what we currently know about the benefits inherent in well-conceived activity programs. Second, we must ensure that children have ample opportunity to participate in meaningful physical activities. Third, the teachers or supervisors of activity programs must become immersed in the attempt to change present levels of motor behavior and fitness. The final step is to determine which procedures and activities produce the expected outcomes.

Indicators of quality secondary school programs

Because of varying backgrounds, personalities, and interests, students should be exposed to a variety of ways to improve fitness, with increasing individual responsibility for deciding which activities they will employ. Competition continues as part of the program, but is not used to exclude continued participation in activities, nor is winning overemphasized.

Providing information, testing, and supervised fitness activities for educational colleagues and the community is also an important ingredient of the physical education program in the secondary schools. The public schools remain the best vehicle for providing programs for positive health for all citizens with television as a potentially powerful ally. Private and commercial fitness programs will only be available to portions of our society, and their personnel are often inadequately educated.

Although no aspect of education is ideally funded, there are two major problems in the promotion of positive health through the schools—the lack of widespread resources for professionals in elementary school physical education and the disproportionate use of physical education/athletic personnel and funds for a small percent of elite performers. Appropriate fitness funding will include personnel, time, facilities, equipment, and other support including daily participation in a fitness program for the entire school.

An effective secondary school program would include students learning the fitness goals and the rationale for them. Learning why different tests and activities are recommended is an essential aspect of the educational fitness program (Franks, 1984). Students would increasingly set their own goals and design activities to enhance healthy behaviors and discontinue unhealthy ones.

Physical activity aims at increased cardiorespiratory function, decreased body fat, flexibility, muscular strength and endurance, good nutrition, rest, ability to cope with stressors of all types, and a life free from harmful substances (e.g., tobacco, alcohol, drugs) would be included, according to Franks. Basic elements of behavior modification would be learned and practiced.

Commitment to Program

Program administrators should now utilize the developed support materials packet with all instructional staff at the department, school, and district level to enlist unanimous commitment to the physical fitness program. Administrators should schedule meetings with various groups including classroom teachers, physical education instructors, principals, school counselors, school nurses, district curriculum staff, and district administrators. The meetings should emphasize commitment to the following points:

- Physical fitness is an important component of the total physical education program and must be well planned in order to meet the needs of all children.
- Physical fitness is a part of total fitness.
- Physical fitness consists of many components each of which is specific in nature.
- Cardiovascular fitness, muscular endurance, strength, body composition, and flexibility may be considered the health-related aspects of physical fitness.
- Power, speed, agility, coordination, balance, and reaction time contribute to one's ability to perform skills and to participate in enjoyable leisure-time activities.
- Physical fitness is important to optimal health.
- Physical fitness contributes to positive physical health.
- Physical fitness contributes to positive mental health.
- Physical fitness is the basis for dynamic and creative activity.
- Physical fitness needs depend upon the individual.

Support for Program

The most important task for the administrator is to obtain necessary support to institute and carry on the program. Arrange for a presentation at one of the regular school governing board meetings. The presentation should focus on what type of program you want and why it is important. Utilize the support packet of written and audiovisual materials developed. Additional support for the program could also come from various community groups or agencies such as parent-teacher organizations, service clubs, the medical profession, and health connected organizations.

It is sometimes more affective to gain support for a school physical fitness program when an outside professional organization or agency is helping to carry your message. Local medical groups have tremendous impact on the public when discussing the role regular exercise plays in reducing risk factors associated with coronary heart disease. Program administrators need to become active members in various community health organizations such as the local heart and lung associations. Presentations to local medical groups outlining your physical fitness program and program needs should be arranged. All community health groups need to hear the message that we are concerned with declining physical fitness test scores, lack of required physical education programs at both the elementary and secondary levels, and lack of resources to conduct quality programs. Here, it is important to emphasize the following:

- Physical fitness contributes to the health, wellness, and productivity of school-age children.
- Physical fitness contributes toward higher academic achievement.
- Lack of exercise is among several factors that contribute to the development of coronary heart disease.
- Physical fitness is an observable and measurable benefit of exercise and sports.
- Physical fitness promotes more disciplined behavior.
- Physical fitness decreases the susceptibility to stress.

References

Albinson, J. G. and Andrews, G. M. 1976. *Child in Sport and Physical Activity.* Baltimore: University Park Press.

Bar-Or, O. 1983. *Pediatric Sports Medicine for the Practitioner.* New York: Springer-Veriag.

Corbin, C. B. and Fletcher, P. 1968. Diet and activity patterns of obese and nonobese elementary school children. *Research Quarterly* 39(4): 922.

Corbin, et al. 1981. *Concepts in Physical Education.* Dubuque: Brown Company Publishers.

Franks, B. D. 1984. Physical fitness in secondary education. *Journal of Physical Education, Recreation and Dance* 55(9): 41-43.

Gilliam, T. B. et. al. 1982. Exercise programs for children: a way to prevent heart disease? *The Physician and Sports Medicine* 10(9): 96-108.

Hayes, A. 1984. Youth physical fitness hearings. *Journal of Physical Education, Recreation and Dance* 55(9): 29-32.

Krahenbuhl, G. S. and Pangrazi, R. P. 1983. Characteristics associated with running performance in young boys. *Medicine and Science in Sports* 15(6): 486-490.

Pangrazi, R. and Slaughter, M. 1984. National youth fitness conference. *Journal of Physical Education, Recreation and Dance* 55(9): 44-46.

Pestolesi, B. 1985. *Physical Education: A Lifetime Commitment.* (Slide/tape promotional packet). AAHPERD Southwest District.

Preliminary Summary of Youth Fitness Hearings Testimony. June 1984. Washington, D.C.: President's Council on Physical Fitness and Sports.

Rarick, L. G. ed. 1973. *Physical Activity, Human Growth, and Activity.* New York: Academic Press.

Rose, K. 1973. *Journal of the American College Health Association* 22:80.

Saltin, B. and Grimby, G. Physiological analysis of middle-aged and old former athletes, comparison with still active athletes of the same ages. *Circulation* 38(6): 1104.

Seefeldt, V. 1984. Physical fitness in preschool and elementary school-aged children. *Journal of Physical Education, Recreation and Dance* 55(9):33-37.

Summary of Findings From National Children and Youth Fitness Study. 1984. Washington, D.C.: Office of Disease Prevention and Health Promotion, U.S. Public Health Service, Department of Health and Human Services.

Wilmore, J. H. and McNamara, J. J. 1974. Prevalance of coronary heart disease risk factors in boys 8 to 12 years of age. *Journal of Pediatrics* 84:4.

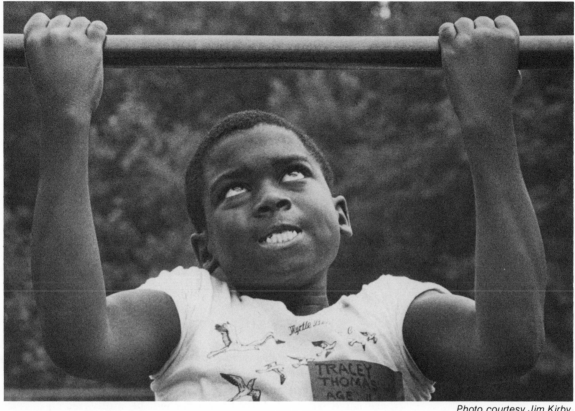

Photo courtesy Jim Kirby.

MANAGEMENT STAGE

3.0

PHYSICAL FITNESS PROGRAM PLANNING

Includes suggested program planning steps, sample philosophy, goals, student objectives, grade level learning experiences, and program activities for a physical fitness program.

**Management
Objective**

**Management
Objective
3.1**

> ## Develop a Physical Fitness Program As a Part of the Total Physical Education Curriculum
>
> ### Management Planning Steps:
>
> Step One   Develop a philosophy statement for your physical fitness program.
>
> Step Two   Develop goals for your physical fitness program.
> Step Three Develop concepts for your physical fitness program.
>
> Step Four   Develop student objectives, suggested learner experiences, and program activities.
>
> Step Five   Develop physical fitness program guidelines.

Sample Physical Fitness Curriculum

**Philosophy of
Physical Fitness**

A physical fitness program for children and youth is one that provides specifically designed physical activities for adequate growth, development, and efficient body functions. It provides information related to these activities so that young people will be motivated to develop optimum fitness and maintain it throughout life. Physical fitness is an important component of the physical education program and should be a part of each daily lesson. The broad range of student interests and abilities are met by quality physical fitness programs which include a wide variety of activities and options.

**Goals of
Physical Fitness**

The goals of a meaningful fitness program are as follows:

- To improve and maintain cardiorespiratory efficiency through aerobic activities, performed on a regular basis, which have sufficient duration and intensity to raise the pulse rate to achieve a training effect.

- To improve and maintain the ability of the muscles to exert force through specific progressive and gradual resistance activities which overload a muscle group.

- To improve and maintain the ability of muscle groups to persist in physical activity, without undue fatigue, by working against a resistance for increasing periods of time.

- To improve and maintain the functional capacity of specific muscles and joints by increasing their full range of motion through static stretching techniques.

- To improve and maintain the relative percentage of lean body mass and fat mass through a conscientious program regulating caloric consumption and expenditures.

- To learn the principles, mechanics, and concepts of all the physical fitness and wellness components as they relate to personal health and physical performance.

With the emphasis that has been placed on physical fitness, there has developed a need to incorporate a conceptual approach which would provide physical education students with an understanding of physical fitness and its relationship to a lifestyle of health-related fitness activities. If our students are to understand physical fitness and to be expected to continue lifelong fitness activities, the program must include the teaching of physical fitness concepts.

General physical fitness:

- Cardiorespiratory endurance, muscular endurance, strength, flexibility and body composition are health-related aspects of physical fitness.

- In order to attain maximal benefits from exercise, it is essential that a regular progressive program be planned to meet the specific needs of the individual.

- There are correct and incorrect ways to exercise and reduce. For maximum benefits, one should know the difference between the facts and the fallacies.

Cardiorespiratory endurance:

- Maintenance of life depends upon the capacity of the heart, blood vessels, and lungs to deliver nutrients and oxygen to your body tissue.

- Cardiorespiratory endurance (aerobic capacity) is increased by working for sufficiently long periods of time at adequate intensity.

- Lack of physical activity is related to cardiorespiratory disease.

Muscular strength and endurance:

- Adequate muscular strength and muscular endurance can contribute to increased work performance, increased resistance to muscle injury and soreness, improved posture, and a general state of good health.

- Strength and muscular endurance is improved by progressively increasing resistance and repetitions.

- Adequate muscular strength and muscular endurance can contribute to increased work performance, increased resistance to muscle injury and soreness, improved posture, and a general state of good health.

Flexibility:

- Flexibility can be improved by increasingly stretching body parts through a full range of motion and sustaining the stretch.

- If you stretch a muscle beyond its normal length an injury can occur.

Body composition:

- Optimal levels of body fat vs. lean body mass (body composition) is related to the attainment of health and a positive self-image.

- An increase in body fat occurs when caloric intake exceeds caloric expenditure.

Physical Fitness Concepts

Sample concepts

Neuromuscular:

- Skills are specific. Because of inherited characteristics, it is normal for persons to find that initially they are good in some physical activities and not so good at others. However, nearly all skills can be improved with appropriate practice.

- Neuromuscular fitness is the aspect of fitness that is concerned with the functioning of the brain and central nervous system and how they control the contractions of muscles that move parts of the body. Some of the components of neuromuscular fitness are: power, agility, coordination, balance, and speed.

Student Objectives and Suggested Learner Experiences

The student objectives and suggested learner experiences that follow are examples only. Program planners will need to refer to the variety of physical fitness program activities listed on page 00 in developing objectives for a total program.

Cardiorespiratory Endurance

Psychomotor Area	Cognitive Area

STUDENT OBJECTIVES

The student will score at or above the 50th percentile on a standardized physical fitness test item which measures cardiorespiratory endurance such as the one mile run, one and one-half mile run, 12 minute walk/run.	The student will answer at a success rate of 75% or better questions which measure concepts of cardiorespiratory endurance.

SUGGESTED GRADE LEVEL EXPERIENCES

Primary—

Runs, jumps, and hops effectively in appropriate games, relays, stunts, and rhythm activities.	Explains why the heart beats faster during exercise and activity.

Intermediate—

Runs a course around the playground, increasing the distance covered each week.	Explains how to determine own resting, exercise, and maximum heart rate.

Junior High—

Participates effectively in vigorous individual, dual, and team sports.	Describes the kinds of activities that promote cardiovascular fitness.

Senior High—

Participates in aerobic activities maintaining a required heart rate at an appropriate training level.	Describes the effects of cardiovascular training on the human body.

Muscular Strength and Endurance

Psychomotor Area	Cognitive Area

STUDENT OBJECTIVES

The student will score at or above the 50th percentile on a standardized physical fitness test item which measures muscular strength and endurance such as the pull-up, flexed arm hang, bent knee sit-up.	The student will answer at a success rate of 75% or better questions which measure concepts of muscular strength and endurance.

SUGGESTED GRADE LEVEL EXPERIENCES

Primary—

Supports own weight from overhead apparatus for extended periods of time.	Describes the role of muscles in performing physical activity.

Intermediate—

Shows progress on pre-post test results on recognized physical fitness test items which measure muscular strength/endurance.	Relates the general principles of exercise related to strength.

Junior High—

Selects and performs two exercises for upper body and two exercises for lower body that develop and maintain muscular strength and endurance.	Describes the general principles of exercise and the guidelines for physical fitness related to muscular strength and endurance.

Senior High—

Possesses sufficient muscular strength and endurance to maintain efficient posture, perform work requirements, and meet emergency situations.	Develops a personal weight training program to develop both strength and muscular endurance.

Flexibility

Psychomotor Area	Cognitive Area

STUDENT OBJECTIVES

The student will score at or above the 50th percentile on a standardized physical fitness test item which measures flexibility such as the sit and reach.	The student will answer at a success rate of 75% or better questions which measure concepts of flexibility.

SUGGESTED GRADE LEVEL EXPERIENCES

Primary—

Moves arms and legs in a full range of motion during dance, stunts, and tumbling.	Explains why stretching the body slowly in various directions is good for you.

Intermediate—

Performs at a satisfactory level basic stunts and tumbling skills on apparatus and mats.	Identifies basic joints and explains their functions.

SUGGESTED GRADE LEVEL EXPERIENCES
(Continued)

Junior High—

Performs at a satisfactory level on appropriate tests of flexibility.

Explains the difference between ballistic and statis stretching.

Senior High—

Demonstrates three static stretches and identifies the targeted muscles.

Explains the general principles of exercise and the guidelines for physical fitness related to flexibility.

Body Composition

Psychomotor Area	Cognitive Area

STUDENT OBJECTIVES

The student will demonstrate the ability to maintain acceptable percentage of body fat which equals 24 percent for girls and 15 percent for boys.

The student will answer at a success rate of 75% or better questions which measure concepts of body composition.

SUGGESTED GRADE LEVEL EXPERIENCES

Primary—

Relates body needs to food groups.

Intermediate—

Participation by grade level in activities that have high caloric expenditure

Describes various ways of controlling body fat through diet and exercise.

Junior High—

Describes ideal weight and the need to lose fat, rather than lean body tissue when losing weight.

Senior High—

Demonstrates the ability to keep a chart to record daily food intake and exercise output in maintaining an ideal amount of body fat.

Physical Fitness Program Activities

Primary Level

Rope jumping
Stretching exercises
Relaxation techniques
Apparatus play
Dance exercise
Walking
Jogging
Endurance games and relays
Nutrition

Intermediate Level

Rope jumping
Stretching exercises
Relaxation techniques
Resistive exercises
Apparatus play
Course challenges
Jogging
Walking
Endurance games and relays
Nutrition
Dance exercises

Junior High Level

Rope jumping
Interval running
Interval swimming
Conditioning exercises
Relaxation techniques
Body alignment
Fitness trail challenges
Dance exercise
Nutrition
Weight training

Senior High Level

Rope jumping
Stretching exercises
Dance exercise
Relaxation techniques
Weight training
Jogging
Swimming
Cycling
Body alignment
Fitness trail challenges
Nutrition

Physical Fitness Program Guidelines

Guidelines which designate the frequently, intensity, and duration of an exercise program must be developed. For exercise to be of benefit students need to exercise at least three times a week. How hard students work depends on their present level of physical fitness. Students should know their fitness target zone and function within that zone. Exercise must be done at least 15 to 30 minutes at one time.

References

Corbin, C. B. and Lindsay, R. L. 1983. *Fitness for Life*. Glenview, IL: Scott Foresman and Company.

Cooperative County Course of Study, Guide to a Balanced Curriculum. 1984. Hayward, CA: Office of the Alameda County Superintendent of Schools.

Physical Education Framework for California Public Schools. 1985. Sacramento: California State Department of Education.

Youth Physical Fitness: 1984. Washington, D.C.: President's Council on Physical Fitness and Sports.

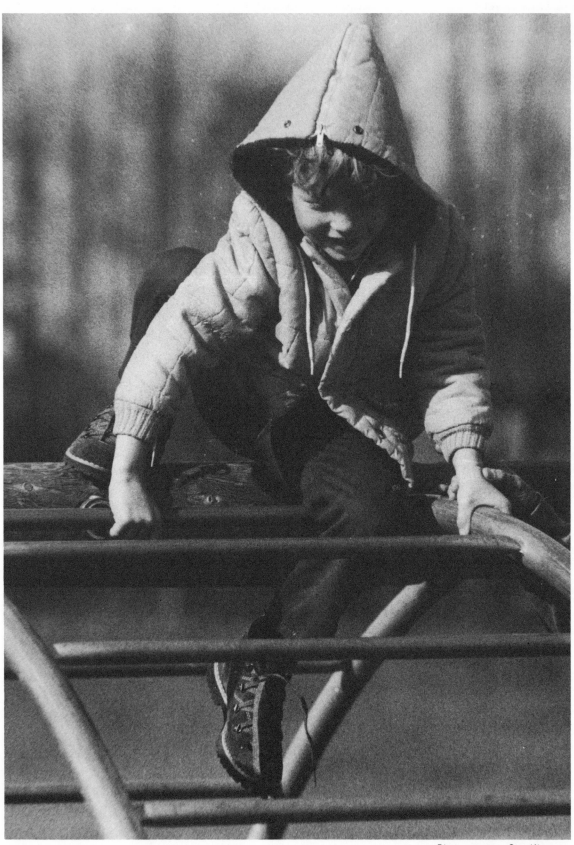

Photo courtesy Sue Klemens.

4.0

PROGRAM IMPLEMENTATION— ADMINISTRATIVE FUNCTIONS

Includes legal provisions, suggested budget process, program staffing criteria, suggested facilities, equipment, supplies, and appropriate instructional materials.

Management Objectives

Management Objective 4.1

Determine the Legal Statutes Which Govern the Physical Fitness Program as Part of Regular Physical Education Instruction

Management Planning Steps:

Step One   Adopt the legal foundations for the physical fitness program based on federal statutes.

Step Two   Adopt the legal foundations for the physical fitness program based on state statutes.

Sample Legal Statutes

Federal Statutes

Title IX, Educational Amendments of 1972, Public Law 92-138. Provides that "no person in the United States shall, on the basis of sex, be excluded from participation in, be denied the benefits of or be subjected to discrimination under any educational program or activity receiving federal financial assistance."

No course may be offered or educational program conducted separately for males or females, including, "health, physical education industrial, business, vocational, technical, home economics, music, and adult education courses."

Physical Education—Separation and Grouping. Students may be separated within physical education classes or activities when engaging in the following sports: wrestling, soccer, football, basketball, and other sports, the purpose or major activity of which involves bodily contact.

Students may be grouped in physical education classes on the basis of ability, provided specified standards of individual performance are utilized. These standards of performance must be applied without regard to sex; however, "where use of a single standard of measuring skill or progress in physical education has an adverse effect on member of one sex ... other appropriate standards which do not have such an effect" shall be used.

Education for All Handicapped Children Act, Public Law 94-142. Provides that every child in a special education program be educated in accordance with individual plans tailored to the child's particular needs and capacities.

"The term 'Special Education' means specially designed instruction, at no cost to parents or guardians, to meet unique needs of a handicapped child, including classroom instruction, instruction in physical education, home instruction, and instruction in hospitals and institutions."

Requires that an individualized education program (or plan) be developed at a meeting of an administrator or designee, the pupil's teacher(s), and, when appropriate, the pupil.

California Education Code, Section 60602. "Physical fitness test" means any test which addresses body structure and composition, and cardiovascular, musculoskeletal, and neuromuscular functions.

"Testing program" means the systematic achievement testing of all pupils in grades 3, 6, 8, 10, 12, and the health-related physical fitness testing of all pupils in any three grades designated by the State Board of Education, required by this chapter in all schools within each school district by means of tests designated by the State Board of Education.

California Education Code, Section 60608. Commencing with the 1986-87 school year, during either the month of March, April, or May, the governing board of each school district maintaining any grade designated by the State Board of Education pursuant to subdivision (c) of Section 60602 shall administer to each pupil in those grades a health-related physical fitness test designated by the Superintendent of Public Instruction. Each physically handicapped pupil and each pupil who is physically unable to take all of the physical fitness test shall be given as much of the test as his or her condition will permit.

Each school district shall submit to its governing board and the State Department of Education the results of its health-related physical fitness testing by July 15 of each year. The department shall compile the results of the annual testing and submit a report by September 15 of each year to the appropriate policy committee of each house of the Legislature for purposes of comparing the performance of California pupils to national norms.

State Statutes

Develop an Operational Budget to Support the Physical Fitness Program

Management Planning Steps:

Step One   Determine the physical fitness budget expenditure classifications and descriptions of each.

Step Two   Determine approximate annual funding necessary for a minimal physical fitness program at each school.

Step Three   Determine approximate annual funding necessary for an expanded physical fitness program at each school.

Management Objective 4.2

Sample Physical Fitness Budget

If minimal funding is not received, program administrators are responsible to implement a physical fitness program using creative and innovative strategies in order to maintain this important component of the physical education curriculum. Budget amounts listed serve only as examples for the categories listed.

Classifications

Classifications	Descriptions
Salaries	
Supervisors Salaries	Consultants, coordinators, supervisors, directors of physical education/physical fitness
Teachers Salaries	Certificated elementary school classroom teachers; elementary school physical education specialists; secondary school physical education instructors
Instructional Aides Salaries	Noncertified physical education/physical fitness aides under the supervision of a teacher
Materials and Supplies	
Student Materials	Physical fitness textbooks, reference books, periodicals, workbooks (all materials used by students)
Teacher Materials	Physical fitness teaching guides, periodicals, magazines, workbooks (all materials used by teachers)
Supplies	Any physical fitness supply item of an expendable nature that is consumed or worn out, deteriorates in use, or easily broken, damaged, or lost such as jump ropes, stop watches, skin calipers
Audiovisual Supplies	Physical fitness motion picture films, filmstrips, television tapes, slides, etc. (some budget classifications include 16mm motion picture films under the equipment category)
Awards	Physical fitness award certificates and patches
Contracted and Support Costs	
Consultants	Physical fitness experts who provide assistance to teachers or pupils in program development
Travel and Conferences	Expenses for employees to travel and attend local, state, district, and national physical education/physical fitness conferences

Classifications	Descriptions
Support Costs	Telephone, postage, printing, data processing services, etc. to support a physical education/physical fitness program
Publicity	Public relations and news media activities to promote the physical education/physical fitness program
Contracts, Rents, Leases	Expenditures for renting or leasing physical fitness equipment or space
Capital Outlay	
Site Development (Outdoor)	Blacktopping, playground markings, playground equipment etc. (all permanently attached to land)
Building Development (Indoor)	Stall bars, climbing ropes, chinning bars, etc. (all permanently attached to buildings)
Equipment	Includes moveable physical fitness equipment of a relatively permanent nature and/or of significant value such as parallel bars, tumbling mats, weight machines

Approximate Annual Funding Necessary for Elementary and Secondary School Physical Fitness Programs

BUDGET CLASSIFICATIONS	MINIMAL FUNDING PROGRAM	SAMPLE COSTS	EXPANDED FUNDING PROGRAM	SAMPLE COSTS
Salaries[1]				
Supervisors Salary	Supervision services provided by principal or district instructional supervisor	None	Supervision services provided by a district physical education supervisor	$(30,000)[2]
Teachers Salary	Instruction provided by regular classroom teachers (elementary)	None	Instruction provided by full-time physical education specialist (elementary)	18,000
	Instruction provided by regular physical education teachers (secondary)		Teacher pupil ratio for individualized fitness Instruction (secondary)	
Instructional Aides Salary	Instructional assistance provided by regular classroom aides (elementary)	None	Instructional assistance provided by trained paraprofessionals in physical fitness (elementary)	5,000
	No instructional aides (secondary)		Employment of instructional aides to hance the physical fitness program (secondary)	
Materials and Supplies				
Student materials (See Management Objective 4.5)	Reference books, periodicals, (one classroom set)	100	Reference books, periodicals (three classroom sets)	300
Teacher materials (See Management Objective 4.5)	Teaching guides, periodicals, magazines (one set per grade level)	200	Teaching guides, periodicals, magazines (one set per teacher)	400
Supplies (See Management Objective 4.4)	Jump ropes, stop watches, skin calipers, etc. (one set per grade level)	500	Jump ropes, stop watches, skin calipers, etc. (two sets per grade level)	1,000
Audiovisual Supplies (See Management Objective 4.4)	Motion picture films, filmstrips, TV tapes, slides, etc.	None	Motion picture films, filmstrips, TV tapes, slides, etc. (one set per school)	2,000[3]

[1] All salaries budgeted will depend on local salary schedules.

[2] Cost for supervisor of physical education usually covered under the district support staff budget.

[3] Cost for purchase of audiovisual supplies usually covered under the district's Instructional Materials Center budget category.

BUDGET CLASSIFICATIONS	MINIMAL FUNDING PROGRAM	SAMPLE COSTS	EXPANDED FUNDING PROGRAM	SAMPLE COSTS
Awards (See Management Objective 5.7)	Physical fitness awards, certificates, and patches for students scoring at the 85th percentile on AAHPERD Youth Fitness Test	50	Physical fitness awards, certificates, and patches for students scoring at the 50th and 85th percentiles on AAHPERD Youth Fitness Test	100
Contracted and Support Costs				
Consultants	None	None	A physical fitness expert is contracted with to consult in program development	500
Travel and Conferences	Travel and attendance for selected staff to one local and one state physical fitness conference	250	Travel and attendance for selected staff to one local, state, and district conference	500
Support Costs	Telephone, postage, printing	150	Telephone, postage, printing, data processing services	300
Publicity	None	None	Public relations and new media activities	100
Contracts, Rents, Leases	None	None	One microcomputer rental or leasing	300
Capital Outlay[4]				
Site Development (See Management Objective 4.4)	Blacktopping, playground markings, or playground equipment, etc.	250	Blacktopping, playground marking, or playground equipment, etc.	500
Building Development (See Management Objective 4.4)	Stall bars, climbing ropes, chinning bars, etc.	250	Stall bars, climbing ropes, chinning bars, etc.	500
Equipment (See Management Objective 4.4)	Tumbling mats, balance beams, parallel bars, etc.	250	Tumbling mats, balance beams, parallel bars etc.	500
TOTALS		2,000		30,000

[4]Major capital outlay items should be budgeted on a five-year plan. Costs listed are for add-on equipment not new construction.

**Management
Objective
4.3**

Staff the School or Department with Credentialed Teachers Qualified to Teach the Concepts and Practices of Physical Fitness to All Students as Part of a Regular Physical Education Program

Management Planning Steps:

Step One   Specify the strengths necessary related to biological, psychological, and sociological foundations.

Step Two   Specify the strengths necessary related to instruction.

Step Three   Specify the strengths necessary related to measurement and evaluation.

Step Four   Specify the strengths necessary related to organization and administration.

Sample Qualifications for Physical Fitness Instructors

**Biological,
Psychological, and
Sociological
Foundations**

- Demonstrate knowledge and understanding regarding functional human anatomy, particularly musculo-skeletal structural characteristics, as applied to movement analysis and design, and to the analysis of motor skills.

- Demonstrate knowledge and understanding regarding immediate, as well as long term, physiological responses which the body experiences as a result of exercise.

- Demonstrate ability to design and conduct instructional programs in accordance with essential physiological considerations and principles.

- Demonstrate competency in communicating the physiological benefits and values to be derived from regular physical activity.

- Demonstrate ability to interpret and apply research findings in exercise physiology to the instructional program.

- Identify and demonstrate understanding of the components of physiological and motor fitness.

- Demonstrate knowledge and understanding of anatomical and physiological deviations in the human organism and the effects on motor performance.

- Demonstrate knowledge and understanding of the social learnings involved through physical activity and its effect on personality, perception, and motivation.

- Demonstrate understanding of the relationship between participation in physical activities and self-realization.

- Demonstrate knowledge and understanding of the relationship of personality dynamics and participation in physical activities.

Instruction

- Demonstrate knowledge and understanding of standardized tests utilized to measure physical and motor fitness.
- Identify performance/instructional objectives which lead to the fulfillment of the goals of physical fitness.
- Demonstrate knowledge of physical fitness developmental activities.
- Demonstrate knowledge of the principles of exercise, various teaching styles, and a variety of instructional approaches available to teaching physical fitness.
- Demonstrate understanding of the importance of personal hygiene, posture, and nutrition to personal well-being.
- Identify the role of physical activity in dynamic living and its contribution to health and the worthy use of leisure time.

Measurement and Evaluation

- Clarify student expectations and evaluation methods at the beginning of each instructional unit.
- Provide students with opportunities to establish goals and evaluate their own results.
- Utilize early assessment data to determine appropriate student outcomes, instructional starting points, and grouping approaches.
- Provide students with early personal assessments and evaluations so that they may make the necessary adjustments to improve their performance.
- Reduce threatening situations by providing sufficient instruction and practice time before evaluation.
- Emphasize individualized instruction that enhances full participation toward the achievement of personal fitness goals.
- Design additive rather than subtractive records and keep them up-to-date and open to learner review.
- Recognize progress when it occurs and allow learners to achieve at different rates of speed.

Organization and Administration

- Identify and demonstrate a knowledge of appropriate student supplies, teachers supplies, facilities, and equipment necessary for conducting a physical fitness program.
- Demonstrate the ability to establish class routines and procedures that will enhance instruction for optimal physical fitness development.

Management Objective 4.4

Provide for Facilities and Equipment That Will Enhance the Physical Fitness Component

Management Planning Steps:

Step One   Survey existing indoor and outdoor physical fitness facilities.

Step Two   Survey existing outdoor and indoor physical fitness equipment.

Step Three   Set priorities and strategies for acquisition of new physical fitness facilities and equipment.

Suggested Facilities and Equipment

Indoor and Outdoor Facilities

Most school budgets classify physical fitness facilities under capital outlay expenditures as follows: outdoor facilities (site development) normally include field areas, hardcourt areas, apparatus areas, running tracks, etc.; indoor facilities (building development) include classrooms, gymnasia, dance rooms, and exercise rooms.

The following outdoor and indoor facilities suggested are for a comprehensive physical education program. Not all listed facilities are required for specific improvement of physical fitness; however, they are needed to facilitate motor and sports skill acquisition which, in turn, will result in improved fitness.

Elementary School Outdoor Facilities for Student Enrollment of 600

Type of facility	Kindergarten	Primary	Middle
		Number Suggested	
Field area 90' × 120'	1	2	
Hardcourt area 60' × 75'	1	4	
Apparatus area (3200 sq. ft.)	1	3	3
Field area 180' × 180'			4
Hardcourt area 80' × 100'			4

Secondary School Outdoor Facilities for Student Enrollment of 750 Junior High School and 1500 Senior High School

Type of facility	Junior High School	Senior High School
	Number suggested	
Field area 260′ × 260′	1	1
Field area 260′ × 460′		1
Hardcourt area 100′ × 100′	3	3
Hardcourt area 100′ × 120′	3	6
Field area 360′ × 360′	1	1
Field area 330′ × 750′	1	1
Apparatus area (1000 sq. ft.)	3	5

Elementary and Secondary School Indoor Facilities

Type of facility	Elementary School	Secondary School
Classrooms	X	X
Auditorium, cafeteria, multi-purpose room	X	
Gymnasium	(Highly recommended)	X
Adapted room		X
Dance studio		X
Dance studio		X
Combination room		X
Weight training room		X
Storage rooms	X	X
Shower and locker rooms		X
Swimming pool		X

Permanent or portable physical fitness equipment of significant value such as weight machines, tumbling mats, or playground equipment are considered capital outlay items. The following indoor and outdoor equipment items are basic to student physical fitness development.

Permanent or Portable Equipment

Elementary School Outdoor Equipment

Kindergarten	Primary	Middle
Climbing structure	Climbing structure	Climbing poles/ropes
Crawling structure	Graduated horizontal bars	Climbing structure
Horizontal travel structure	Horizontal travel structure	Graduated horizontal bars
Low turning bar	Low turning bar	Horizontal ladder
Swing rings	Swing rings	Parallel bars
Tire swings	Tire swings	Swing rings
		Tire swings

Secondary School Outdoor Equipment

Junior High School	Senior High School
Climbing poles/ropes	Climbing poles/ropes
Graduated horizontal bars	Graduated horizontal bars
Parallel bars	Parallel bars
Horizontal ladders	Horizontal ladders
Vaulting bars	Vaulting bars

Note: Outdoor permanent equipment could be located in one central location for individualized or circuit training. If space is available, the equipment may be spaced over an extended area to form a fitness trail. Additional equipment such as scaling walls, turning posts, and directional signs may be added to expand the fitness trail at minimal cost.

Elementary and Secondary School Indoor Equipment

Elementary	Secondary	
Adjustable vaulting box	Abdominal board	Weights
Parallel bars	Climbing ropes	Weight machines
Horizontal bars	Horizontal bars	Rings
Stegel	Parallel bars	Tumbling mats
Tumbling mats	Peg boards	Exercise bicycle
Homemade weights	Indoor jogger	Rowing machine

Priorities and Strategies for Acquiring Facilities and Equipment

Most school budgets do not include funds to acquire physical fitness facilities such as gymnasiums, exercise rooms, or hardcourt areas. Very seldom do schools add on to existing sites and buildings due to extreme cost in construction. If program administrators determine a facility deficiency, and are unable to carry on an adequate physical fitness program, a school site and building improvement plan should be developed or a local long-term fund-raising campaign should be organized.

Facilities

Priority for program administrators in acquiring physical fitness facilities should be on new school construction. In most states, a percentage of new school construction funds are allocated for site and building development. All new site and building construction plans should include appropriate outdoor and indoor physical fitness facilities.

Equipment

Most outdoor or indoor physical fitness equipment is expensive. Program administrators will need to carefully review the equipment survey results, study equipment suggestions provided, and set priorities for new acquisitions. Physical fitness equipment requires capital outlay and will necessitate considerable justification for purchase. School and district administrators, business office directors, and maintenance supervisors need to be included in the acquisition process.

There are several physical fitness equipment companies willing to send you their catalogs with current price lists. Equipment company sales representatives exhibit at state, district, and national conferences and have current information on new products.

School parent-teacher organizations should be approached for financial assistance in acquiring outdoor physical fitness equipment. Local service clubs are also interested in projects which involve high visibility such as participating in actual installation of a physical fitness trail or challenge courses.

Provide Appropriate Instructional Materials and Supplies for Effective Instruction

Management Planning Steps:

Step One   Survey available instructional materials, audiovisual aids, and program supplies.

Step Two   Establish priorities for purchase of instructional materials, audiovisual aids, and program supplies.

Step Three   Arrange for program implementation of the materials and supplies.

Management Objective 4.5

Sample Instructional Materials, Audiovisual Aids, and Program Supplies

The following materials and supplies are only samples of available resources for physical fitness instruction. Each program administrator should regularly send for, review, and purchase materials and supplies for teacher inservice orientation and utilization.

Instructional Materials

Student emphasis

- *Fitness for Life*, 2nd Edition, Charles B. Corbin and Ruth Lindsey, Scott Foresman and Company, 1900 East Lake Avenue, Gleview, Illinois, 60025 (Secondary level)

- Have a Healthy Heart program, 4095 173rd Place, Southwest, Bellevue, Washington, 98008 (Elementary Level)

- Fitness Finders materials, 133 Teft Road, Spring Arbor, Michigan, 49283 (Elementary and Secondary Level)

- Superheart program, Lucy Stroble, Project Director, P.O. Box 2000, SUNY at Cortland, Cortland, New York, 13045

- Childrens Health International program, Dennis Estabrook, Director, P.O. Box 3100, Manhattan Beach, California, 90266

- Chicago Heart Health Curriculum Program, Chicago Heart Association, 20 North Wacker Drive, Chicago, Illinois, 60606 (Elementary and Secondary Level)

- Health Activities Project, Hubbard Company, P.O. Box 104, Northbrook, Illinois, 60062
- It's Fun to be Fit for Life Program, P.O. Box 14312, Dayton, Ohio, 45414
- *Young Runners Handbook*, Kinney Shoe Corporation, 233 Broadway, New York, New York, 10007

Teacher emphasis

- Walt Disney Educational Media Company, 500 S. Buena Vista St., Burbank, California, 91521
- Fitness Finders materials, 133 Teft Road, Spring Arbor, Michigan, 49283
- Your Local American Heart Association or The National Center of the American Heart Association, 7320 Greenville Avenue, Dallas, Texas, 75231
- Sunflower Project, Shawnee Mission Public Schools, Mohawk Instructional Center, 6649 Lamar, Shawnee Mission, Kansas, 66202
- *Teach for Fitness*, A manual for teaching fitness concepts for K-12 physical education, Laurie Priest, Eric Clearing House on Teacher Education, One Dupont Circle, Suite 610, Washington, D.C. 20026
- *Health and Fitness Through Physical Activity*, Michael Pollock, Jack Wilmore, and Samuel Fox III, John Wiley and Sons, New York, 1978
- *Rating the Exercise*, Charles T. Kontzleman and the editors of Consumer Guide, William Morrow and Company, Inc., 1978, 105 Madison Ave., New York, New York 10016
- "How Different Sports Rate in Promoting Physical Fitness," C. Carson Conrad, reprint from *Medical Times*, 80 Shore Rd., Port Washington, New Mexico, 11050
- *The New Aerobics*, Kenneth Cooper, 1975, Bantam Books, New York
- *Fitness for Every Body*, Linda Garrison and Ann Read, Mayfield Publishing Co., 1980, Palo Alto, California
- "Cardiovascular Fitness Education for Elementary Students," David Jenkins, from the *Journal of Physical Education and Recreation*, 49 (5):59; May 1978. (ERIC No. EJ 187 830)
- "Fun in Fitness at the Elementary School Level," James G. Johnston, from the *Canadian Association for Health, Physical Education and Recreation Journal*, 46 (2):28-37, March-April 1980
- "Jogging Through the Circulatory Systems," Kathleen Kern in the *New York State Association for Health, Physical Education, and Recreation Journal* 31(2):8-9; Fall 1980
- "Teaching Physical Fitness: An Action Approach," Karen King, in *Health Education* 12 (1): 34; January-February 1981

Audiovisual Aids

- Walt Disney Educational Media Company: *Fitness and Me* Series, K-3 (3 films); *Fun to be Fit* Series, 4-6 (3 films); *Fit to be You* Series, 7-9 (3 films); *Fitness for Living* Series, 10-12 (3 films)
- *Why Exercise*, Associated Film Service
- *Physical Fitness—The New Perspective*, Sterling Educational Films

- *Run ... For Your Life*, Sterling Educational Films
- *Run Dick, Run Jane*, Brigham Young University
- *Weight Training for Everybody*, Universal Educational and Visual Arts
- *Strength Training for Women Athletes*, Focus Film Productions
- *What's Good to Eat*, Perennial Education, Inc.

Program Supplies

Balls of various sizes	Cageball	Jump ropes
Flexibility testing box	Hoops	Scooter boards (elementary only)
Stop watches	Tape measures	Wands
Tug-of-war rope	Scales	Medicine ball (secondary only)
Skin calipers	Flying disks	Parachutes (elementary only)

Establishing priorities for purchase

Based on the survey of all materials and supplies available in classrooms, educational libraries, multi-media centers, and resource centers related to physical fitness, establish a priority for purchase. Purchase requests should reflect a balance between instructional materials and supplies. The fitness goals are greatly enhanced when available instructional materials and supplies are provided for the instructional program.

Program implementation

Program managers should regularly schedule and conduct staff inservice sessions related to the implementation of instructional materials in the classroom. A plan should be developed in cooperation with district instructional material center staff for effective distribution of materials. Maintenance, repair, and replacement of program supplies are also considerations for the administrator in program implementation.

References

Coates, E. and Flynn, R. 1979. *Planning Facilities for Athletics, Physical Education, and Recreation.* Reston, VA: American Alliance of Health, Physical Education, Recreation, and Dance.

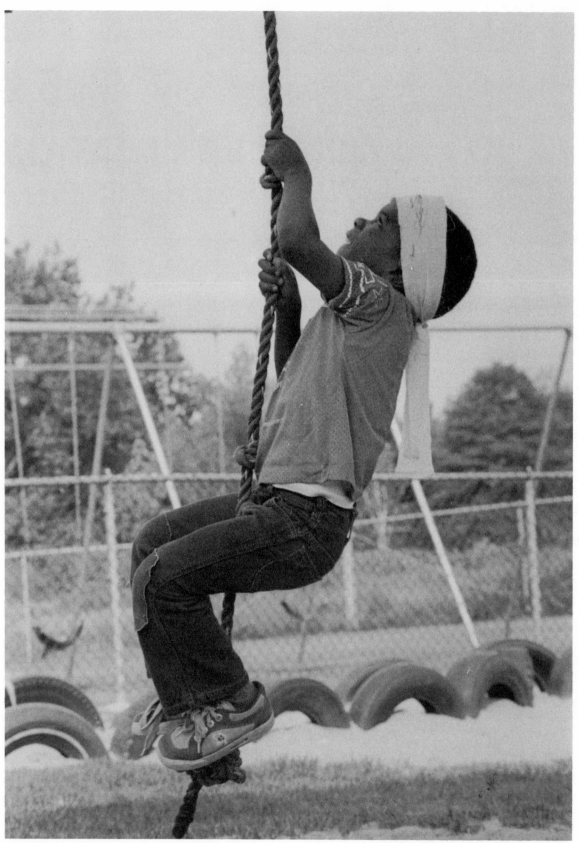

Photo courtesy Carolyn Carlson.

5.0

PROGRAM IMPLEMENTATION INSTRUCTIONAL FUNCTIONS

Includes suggested instructional functions including test selection, computer utilization, test administration, and utilizing program and professional support activities, and a plan to provide for students and staff incentive.

Management Objectives

Management Objective 5.1

Establish a Physical Fitness Testing Program That Will Assess the Physical Fitness Level of All Students

Management Planning Steps:

Step One   Determine if your state department of education or legislature mandates a statewide physical fitness test.

Step Two   Select a recognized national test battery or approved test items if your state does not mandate a test.

Sample Physical Fitness Testing Program

Mandated State Testing

Some states, including California, South Carolina, and Texas, have mandated statewide physical fitness testing programs which require testing in all or designated grades. Some require districts to report results of test scores for statewide study which provides each school with a comparison to state norms.

Comparing test scores with local norms should give a closer-to-home comparison of each students physical fitness level assuming local norms are developed from a sampling of both sexes and all ages throughout the school or district. Comparing test scores nationally will certainly give your school or district more credibility. However, if you don't use a national test, you can't compare with national norms. Therefore, if a state mandated testing program does not exist, is suggested that schools or districts use a national test. There are in existence computer programs which will compare your national test scores with local, state, and national norms (see Management Objective 5.2). Schools or districts not wanting to use a national test could develop their own local test, local norms, and computer programs to process test scores.

Selecting a National Test Battery or Approved Test Items

General Considerations

- Test items should measure the present physical fitness level of all students as stated in the curriculum goals and student objectives.
- Tests should measure a developmental area which extends from severely limited dysfunction to high levels of functional capacity; the test battery should be applicable to boys and girls ages six to eighteen.
- Tests should be administered, scored, and interpreted by teachers with a limited knowledge of physical fitness and test components.
- The test battery should require a minimum of student testing time and specific supplies and equipment.

- Cardiorespiratory endurance—the ability of the body system to maintain efficient production and distribution of energy needs and removal of exercise waste products
- Muscular strength—the ability of a muscle to exert a force or move a particular heavy weight one time
- Muscular endurance—the ability of a muscle to repeat many times an activity which requires a level of strength
- Flexibility—the ability to move a particular joint in the body through its full range of motion
- Body composition—the make-up of the body in lean body mass or weight (muscle, bone, needed tissues, and organs) and in fat mass or weight

**Physical Fitness
Psychomotor
Components**

- Agility—changing of direction quickly
- Power—using skills requiring strength and quick moves
- Speed—moving fast

**Motor Fitness (skill)
Components**

Cardiorespiratory endurance:
- 1 mile run
- 1½ mile run
- 1 mile walk
- 12 min. jog or walk

Muscle strength/endurance:
- upper arm—chin-up, pull-up, flexed arm hang
- abdomen—bent knee sit-up
- leg—standing long jump, vertical jump

Flexibility:
- sit and reach

Body composition:
- skin fold
- body mass index

Agility:
- shuttle run

Power:
- standing long jump
- vertical jump

Speed:
- 50 yard dash
- 100 yard dash

**Some Test Items
Which Measure
Each Component**

Sample Test Questions to Assess Muscular Strength and Endurance Concept

Concept—Adequate muscular strength and muscular endurance can contribute to increased work performance, increased resistance to muscle injury and soreness, improved posture, and a general state of good health.

Grade Level	Taxonomy	Sample Questions
Elementary	Focus: Knowledge Indicators: Simple recall, one simple, isolated fact, truth	Muscles are fastened to other parts of the body by: a. bones b. ligaments c. tendons d. none of these Muscle strength is: a. the ability to move a heavy weight once b. the ability to play sports c. the ability to life weights d. the ability to move something many times Muscle endurance is: a. the ability to move a heavy weight once b. the ability to play sports c. the ability to lift weights d. the ability to move something many times
Junior High School	Focus: Understanding Indicators: Comprehension, why, two or more facts, breaking it into parts, applied principle	Muscles usually contract: a. by themselves b. on a signal from the brain c. when they are warm d. when they are cold Specificity to improve muscle strength means: a. exercising a specific muscle b. using a heavy load of weight c. using a light load of weight d. exercising every day Which two of these activities can help build muscle strength for most boys and girls? a. sit-ups b. playing volleyball c. rope climbing d. shooting baskets

Continued

Grade Level	Taxonomy	Sample Questions
Senior High School	Focus: Application Indicators: Value judgements, synthesis, analysis, evaluation, choice, lifestyle	Which of these statements is not accurate? a. few people require muscle strength b. muscle strength in some parts of the body relates directly to health c. muscle strength and muscle endurance are closely related d. performing 15 pull-ups demonstrates only muscle strength How often should you train with weights? a. daily b. two days a week c. once a week d. every other day A friend wants to develop strength, what type of exercise would probably be best? a. isotonic exercises b. stretching exercises c. only grip and leg exercises d. sign up for track

Sample Test Questions to Assess Flexibility Concept

Concept — Flexibility can be improved by increasingly stretching body parts through a full range of motion and sustaining the stretch

Grade Level	Taxonomy	Sample Questions
Elementary	Focus: Knowledge Indicators: Simple recall, one simple, isolated fact, truth	Muscles and other connecting tissues should be stretched a. once a week b. only after running c. every day d. only when it is cold The best stretching exercises are those done a. slowly b. quickly c. after exercise d. in water Body joints are held together mostly by which two structures? a. ligaments b. skin c. muscles d. nerves

Continued

Grade Level	Taxonomy	Sample Questions
Junior High School	Focus: Understanding Indicators: Comprehension, why, two or more facts, breaking it into parts, applied principle	Stretching exercises will help a. build strength b. avoid injuries c. burn calories d. none of these The muscle group which should be stretched last is a. the neck muscles b. the side muscles c. the back muscles d. the leg muscles Joints are prepared for vigorous physical activity by a. jogging and weight training b. warm-ups and stretching c. rope climbing and sit-ups d. push-ups and jumping jacks
Senior High School	Focus: Application Indicators: Value judgements, synthesis, analysis, evaluation, choice, lifestyle	To overload a muscle for the flexibility part of fitness you must a. circle the track one extra time b. lift as heavy a weight as you can each time you lift c. stretch the muscle farther than it is normally stretched d. stretch less than you normally should Threshold of training for flexibility applies to a. both active and passive stretching b. only active stretching c. only passive stretching d. neither active nor passive stretching The difference between static flexibility and dynamic flexibility is a. the number of times and speed with which exercise is done b. the specific muscles that are stretched c. the amount of flexibility the person needs d. the kind of strength the person has

Program planners should develop additional questions for each physical fitness component.

AAPHERD Youth Fitness Test Manual 1976 Edition, American Alliance for Health, Physical Education, Recreation, and Dance, 1900 Association Drive, Reston VA 22091

AAHPERD Health Related Physical Fitness Test Manual, 1980, American Alliance for Health, Physical Education, Recreation, and Dance, 1900 Association Drive, Reston, VA 22091

Physical Fitness Testing of the Disabled Project Unique, 1985, Joseph P. Unnick, Francis F. Short, Human Kinetics Publishers, Inc., Box 5076, Champaign, IL 61820

Special Fitness Test Manual for Mentally Retarded Persons, American Alliance for Health, Physical Education, Recreation, and Dance, 1900 Association Drive, Reston VA 22091

National physical fitness test batteries

Incorporate a Computer Assisted Physical Fitness Program to Facilitate Instruction

Management Planning Steps:

Step One   Determine type of physical fitness computer assisted programs (software) needed and compatible with your physical fitness test battery.

Step Two   Purchase or develop physical fitness computer assisted programs to match program needs and type of computers available.

Management Objective 5.2

Sample Computer Programs for Physical Fitness

Information processing and data storage programs can be utilized on either the mainframe or microcomputer. These types of programs are limited in that they only process test scores and produce statistical profiles. Some include normative data ranking, frequency distributions, percentile rankings, parent reports, and comparison of test scores from one testing period to the other. If your program needs can be met by supplying statistical reports only, you will then need to identify what type of report is desired and what hardware is available.

The advantage of a mainframe computer is that it will store more data, handle larger numbers of students, and process information more quickly. The advantage of a microcomputer is greater access, more flexibility, less expensive software, and a wider variety of available programs.

Available Software— Information Processing and Data Storage

Information processing and data storage programs

Program:	Fitnessgram Institute of Aerobics Research 12200 Preston Road Dallas, TX 75230
Computer type:	Mainframe
Printout Sample:	Semester Report
Description:	This report displays all scores—raw scores and derived scores for all students by grade, teacher, school. Test scores are from the AAHPERD Health Related Physical Fitness Test

Physical Education Testing
Semester Report: Spring 1983

Student Name: _____ Teacher: _____

Grade: _____ School: _____

Period: _____ District: _____

Sex	Age Yr-Mo	Height Ft-In	Weight Lbs.	Sit & Reach Cent.	Sit-up	Skinfold (mm) Tricep	Subscapular	Walk/Run Type Min:Sec Yard	Total Score
F	15:04	4-11	68	14 0%	15 5%	8.0 100%	3.0	1 mile 5:46 100%	200
F	14:03	5-01	110	31 40%	36 50%	9.0 85%	7.0	1 mile 10:03 40%	205
F	11:05	5-04	108	26 35%	15 5%	9.5 45%	10.5	1 mile 8:56 80%	190
F	15:00	5-01	101	46 95%	45 80%	10.5 75%	9.5	1 mile 7:54 90%	240

Program:	Physical Performance Testing Procedures Regional Education Data Processing Center San Diego County Office of Education 6401 Linda Vista Road San Diego, CA 92111
Computer type:	Mainframe
Printout Sample:	Physical Performance Test Profile Card
Description:	This report displays the percentile score for each student on a graph-like form. The form makes it possible to indicate the scores achieved per event. Variable number of asterisks are used to represent the percentile score indicated on the graph.

Physical Performance Test Profile Card

STUDENT NAME	GRADE	STUDENT NUMBER	SCHOOL	TESTING PROGRAM	DATE TESTED
	04	3769553	955-632	PPT 74	05-76

TEST	TEST RESULTS	00 01 02 03 04 06 08 10 12 15 18 21 25 29 33 37 42 47 52 57 62 66 70 74 78 81 84 87 89 91 93 95 96 97 98 99
LONG JUMP	40%	★★★★★★★★★★★★★
PULL UP	40%	★★★★★★★★★★★★★★
SIT UP	70%	★★★★★★★★★★★★★★★★★★★★
CHAIR PUSHUP	90%	★★★★★★★★★★★★★★★★★★★★★★★★★★
SIDE STEP	90%	★★★★★★★★★★★★★★★★★★★★★★★★★★
JCG WALK	35%	★★★★★★★★★★★★★
FLEXED ARM		

INDIVIDUAL TEST PROFILE

	1	2	3	4	5	6	7		9
T SCORES	27 29 31 32	34 37 23 24	38 39 41 42	43 44 46 47	48 49 51 52	53 54 56 57	58 59 61 62	63 64 66 67	68 69 71 73+
		BELOW AVERAGE			AVERAGE			ABOVE AVERAGE	

Program: Physical Performance Testing Procedures
Regional Education Data Processing Center
San Diego County Office of Education
6401 Linda Vista Road
San Diego, CA 92111

Computer type: Mainframe
Printout Sample: Frequency Distribution
Description: By computing the statistical information based on the population, event, score data, and displays of frequencies, percentages and percentile of scores by event will be in tabular form. At the bottom of each event are listed the standard deviation, variance, mean, median, standard error of the mean, and first and third quartile computations.

Frequency Distribution Chart

PPT   FORM 74   LEVEL   GRADE 04   BOYS

	LONG JUMP				SIT UP				CHAIR PUSHUP		
RAW SCORE	FREQ. NO.	%AGE TOTAL	PSEUDO %ILE	RAW SCORE	FREQ. NO.	%AGE TOTAL	PSEUDO %ILE	RAW SCORE	FREQ. NO.	%AGE TOTAL	PSEUDO %ILE
33	1	4.5	96	38	1	4.0	96	71	1	4.0	96
32	1	4.5	92	33	1	4.0	92	65	1	4.0	92
28	1	4.5	88	29	1	4.0	88	57	1	4.0	88
25	1	4.5	84	27	1	4.0	84	46	2	8.0	80
24	1	4.5	80	26	1	4.0	80	45	1	4.0	76
20	1	4.5	76	23	1	4.0	76	43	1	4.0	72
18	1	4.5	72	22	1	4.0	72	37	1	4.0	68
17	1	4.5	68	21	1	4.0	68	35	1	4.0	64
16	2	9.1	59	20	1	4.0	64	32	1	4.0	60
15	1	4.5	55	19	2	8.0	56	31	1	4.0	56
14	2	9.1	46	16	2	8.0	48	30	2	8.0	48
13	1	4.5	42	14	1	4.0	44	29	1	4.0	44
12	1	4.5	38	13	2	4.0	40	28	2	4.0	40
11	2	9.1	29	12	2	4.0	36	25	3	12.0	28
10	1	4.5	25	10	3	12.0	24	20	1	4.0	24
9	1	4.5	21	7	1	4.0	20	19	2	8.0	16
6	1	4.5	17	5	1	4.0	16	18	1	4.0	12
5	1	4.5	13	4	1	4.0	12	9	2	8.0	4
4	1	4.5	9								

LONG JUMP		SIT UP		CHAIR PUSHUP	
TOTAL STUDENTS	22	TOTAL STUDENTS	24	TOTAL STUDENTS	25
MEAN = 14.2	MEDIAN = 14.5	MEAN = 14.1	MEDIAN = 16.0	MEAN = 25.6	MEDIAN = 30.0
Q1 = 11.0	Q3 = 20.0	Q1 = 11.0.	Q3 = 22.5	Q1 = 25.0	Q3 = 30.0
STD DEVIATION	10.45	STD DEVIATION	11.51	STD DEVIATION	20.99
VARIANCE	109.27	VARIANCE	132.42	VARIANCE	440.60
STD ERROR MEAN	+/- 2.28	STD ERROR MEAN	+/- 2.40	STD ERROR MEAN	+/- 4.29

Programs that Process Information, Store Data, and Provide Student Activity Recommendations

These types of programs, in addition to processing information and storing data, will provide student activity recommendations to assist the instructor in designing individualized developmental programs based on diagnosed needs. Both mainframes and microcomputers can utilize these programs. Administrators need to identify both software and hardware needs. Be reminded that the microcomputer will give you better access and more software availability.

Sample Programs

Program: Fitnessgram
                Institute of Aerobics Research
                12200 Preston Road
                Dallas, TX 75230

Computer type: Mainframe
Printout Sample: Fitnessgram
Description: The Fitnessgram provides the opportunity for school-age youngsters to receive an individual computerized printout report card comparing their fitness test scores against the established national norms on the AAHPERD Youth Fitness Test and the AAHPERD Health Related Physical Fitness Test. The Fitnessgram also provides a composite fitness score and a prescription statement regarding how to improve or maintain one's current level of fitness.

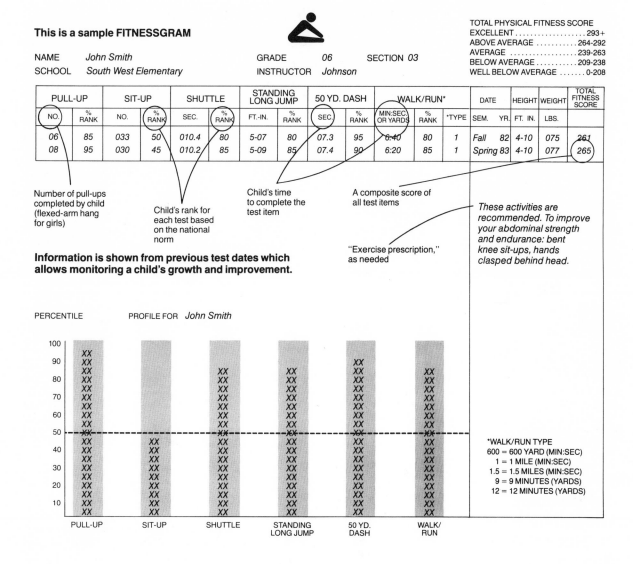

This is a sample FITNESSGRAM

NAME   *John Smith*
SCHOOL   *South West Elementary*

GRADE   *06*   SECTION *03*
INSTRUCTOR   *Johnson*

TOTAL PHYSICAL FITNESS SCORE
EXCELLENT . . . . 293+
ABOVE AVERAGE 264-292
AVERAGE 239-263
BELOW AVERAGE 209-238
WELL BELOW AVERAGE 0-208

PULL-UP		SIT-UP		SHUTTLE		STANDING LONG JUMP		50 YD. DASH		WALK/RUN*			DATE		HEIGHT	WEIGHT	TOTAL FITNESS SCORE
NO.	% RANK	NO.	% RANK	SEC.	% RANK	FT.-IN.	% RANK	SEC.	% RANK	MIN:SEC. OR YARDS	% RANK	*TYPE	SEM.	YR.	FT. IN.	LBS.	
06	85	033	50	010.4	80	5-07	80	07.3	95	6:40	80	1	Fall	82	4-10	075	261
08	95	030	45	010.2	85	5-09	85	07.4	90	6:20	85	1	Spring 83		4-10	077	265

Number of pull-ups completed by child (flexed-arm hang for girls)

Child's rank for each test based on the national norm

Child's time to complete the test item

A composite score of all test items

"Exercise prescription," as needed

These activities are recommended. To improve your abdominal strength and endurance: bent knee sit-ups, hands clasped behind head.

Information is shown from previous test dates which allows monitoring a child's growth and improvement.

PERCENTILE   PROFILE FOR *John Smith*

| | PULL-UP | SIT-UP | SHUTTLE | STANDING LONG JUMP | 50 YD. DASH | WALK/ RUN |

*WALK/RUN TYPE
600 = 600 YARD (MIN:SEC)
1 = 1 MILE (MIN:SEC)
1.5 = 1.5 MILES (MIN:SEC)
9 = 9 MINUTES (YARDS)
12 = 12 MINUTES (YARDS)

Program: National Health Related Physical Fitness Profile
    for Children Ages 6 through 12
    Dr. Sharon Ann Plowman
    1333 Tilton Park Drive
    DeKolb, IL 60115

Computer type: Microcomputer

Printout Sample: National Health Related Physical Fitness Profile
    Ages 6-12

Description: This printout shows test score results and graphs present status for each student. Also suggests developmental play activities for improvement of each component measured.

National Health Related Physical Fitness Profile
for Children Ages 6 through 12

Andy Average   Age: 11

	Distance Run	Skin Fold	Sit- Ups	Sit & Reach
TERRIFIC!				
GETTING THERE!		*		
WORK HARDER!	*		*	
NEED LOTS OF WORK!				*
Test Score	9.55	15.0	35	21
Percentile	35	51	41	21

Your percent body fat is 13.14%

Play activities to help your heart become stronger and your body thinner

Brisk walking
Riding bicycle
Jogging or running
Swimming laps
Rope jumping

To get your heart fit select any of these activities and see if you can perform it for 1 minute without rest. Each day try to add 1 minute to your exercise time.

Exercises to strengthen abdominal muscles

Lay on your back with knees bent

Put hands on thighs, slide hands to knees
Put hands on thighs, slide elbows to knees
Cross arms on chest, sit up

Exercises to improve low-back flexibility

Standing

Slowly bend down and try to touch floor
Cross legs, bend down and try to touch the floor
Spread legs, bend down and reach back through legs
Bend and sway in your various directions

Program: Fitness Appraisal, Inc.
                    P.O. Box 27296
                    San Diego, CA 92129

Computer type: Microcomputer
Printout Sample: Percent Body Fat Program
Description: This printout charts a student's body fat
                    percentage and compares it with the normal
                    range. A weight maintenance program is then
                    prescribed considering data collected.

Percent Body Fat Program

Height-weight tables are not very accurate in determining your ideal body weight. A reliable method is to assess your body fat percentage (what part of your weight is fat). Thus, ideal body weight will be calculated based on your ideal body fat percentage for your age and sex. Your assessment is listed below.

Body Fat Comparison

Your fat %   ★★★★★★★★★★★★★★★

Norm %   ###############

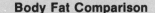

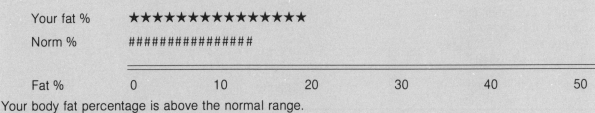

Fat %   0   10   20   30   40   50

Your body fat percentage is above the normal range.
An excellent body fat percentage for young men is 10-14%.

Ideal Body Weight Determination

Your present weight is 120.
Your present percent body fat is 19.1.
You have 23 pounds of fat and 97 pounds of muscle, bone, and water.
Your ideal body fat percentage is 10.

It will take about 6.1 weeks to lose 12.3 pounds of fat.
Your ideal body weight in 6.1 weeks is 109 (includes growth weight).

You should consume 2070 calories a day if you exercise aerobically for 30 minutes a day.
Without exercise you should consume 1770 calories a day.
When you reach your ideal body weight, increase your caloric intake to 2270 at a slow rate.

Some Physical Fitness Programs (software) Available

Note: This is not a complete list. Program planners will need to research state and national computer program catalogs for newly developed programs.

Program	Computer Type		Program Type	
	Mainframe	**Microcomputer**	**Information Processing**	**Program Instruction**
Fitnessgram Institute of Aerobics Research 12200 Preston Road Dallas, Texas	Prime 750	Apple IIe	X	X

Physical Performance
  Testing Procedures
Regional Educational Data
  Processing Center
San Diego County Office of
  Education
6401 Linda Vista Road
San Diego, CA 92111
	Burroughs
	  6900
			X	

Fitness Wellness
  Through Dynamic
  Physical Education K-6
Burgess Publishing
  Company
Minneapolis, MN 55435
		Apple IIe	X	X

National Health Related
  Physical Fitness Profile
  for Children Ages 6-12
  and 13-18 (two programs)
133 Tilton Park Drive
DeKolb, IL 60115
		Apple IIe	X	X

President's Physical Fitness Program Hartley Courseware, Inc. Diamondale, MI 48821		Apple II or IIe TRS 80 Model III	X	

AAHPERD Youth Fitness
  Data Base System
Physical Education/REACT
Minnesota Department of
  Education
550 Cedar
St. Paul, MN 55101
		Apple II	X	

Health Related Fitness Test Gart Spindt Hard High School 24405 Scodeland Drive Newhall, CA 91321		Apple II	X	X

Program	Computer Type		Program Type	
	Mainframe	Microcomputer	Information Processing	Program Instruction
Health Related Test Scoring Arthur Carpet Computek Company 28278 Enderly Canyon Country, CA 91321		Apple IIe	X	X
Physical Evaluation Programs (PEP) Educational Activities, Inc. Freport, NY 11520		Apple II or IIe TRS 80 Model III	X	X
General Fitness Fitness Appraisal, Inc. P.O. Box 27296 San Diego, CA 92129		Apple IIe or TRS 80 Model	X	X
Fitscore Miero-Matics, Inc. P.O. Box 2723 Norman, OK 73070		Any micro with a spread- sheet program	X	

Health Fitness Profile
for Children Ages 6-12
    and
Health Fitness Profile
for Children Ages 13-17
    and
Computer Applications of
Health Related Physical
Fitness Test
    and
Analysis Health Related
Physical Fitness Test
Scores (4 programs)
AAHPERD
1900 Association Drive
Reston, VA 22091
		Apple II, II+,
		IIe
			X	X

Management Objective 5.3

Provide Professional Support to Staff on Test Administration and Utilization of Test Results

Management Planning Steps:

Step One   Consult with staff and conduct staff development on test administration.

Step Two   Consult with staff and conduct staff development on test results utilization.

Sample Test Administration and Utilization

Test Administration

Pretest clearance and general orientation

Ascertain the medical-physical status of all students in your class. Those with medical-physical restrictions should be identified and given explicit instructions concerning the level of participation in the testing program, e.g., excused, involved in a modified testing program, to be tested at a later date, etc. Consultation with school nurse, family physician, or parents may be necessary to clarify the appropriate level of participation for a particular student.

Once the medical-physical disposition of the students has been established and appropriate categorization decided on, a step-wise process of achieving the stated purpose and objectives of the testing program should begin. Special attention should be given to guidelines for physical conditioning and general preparation for the testing program. A realistic plan including organization and scheduling of student test groups, space, time, equipment, and supplies is essential.

Pretest conditioning activities

Most recognized physical fitness test batteries will require the basic abilities of strength, power, agility, flexibility, and endurance. Physical activities that focus on these basic abilities should comprise the core of any physical conditioning regimen used to prepare students for the testing program.

Physical conditioning regimens composed of activities utilizing the criteria of effort, speed, and duration can effect specific development and improvement by the use of the "overload principle." This principle involves a progressive increase in effort, speed, and/or duration over the training period to induce an increase in a specific fitness ability, which in turn is expressed by an improvement in the designated performance test. Routine physical activity—minimum three times per week—and a progressive overload implemented approximately every two to three weeks will result in consistent improvement.

Pretest warm-up activities

All vigorous physical activity should be preceded by five to ten minutes of warm-up exercises. Suggested warm-up activities include walking or easy jogging, followed by a series of static and very slow-speed calisthenics. The series of calisthenics should include exercises for the major joints and limbs of the body. For convenience, the exercise can be categorized for upper body, trunk, and lower body. Each of these anatomical areas should include a static stretch for 30 seconds in two planes of motion e.g., sit-reach and lateral trunk twist, and very slow dynamic exercise of the principal joints e.g., side leg raises or hip flexors.

Students should be organized in small groups (three to six per group) and rotated as a group from one test station to the other. This grouping scheme can be used to place individuals of like ability together to promote competitive effort. Since the testing program is designed to assess maximal performance, this arrangement may serve to motivate students to perform at their best; in contrast, the poorer students will not feel intimidated if the competition is more evenly arranged. It is also wise to place one student of some leadership ability with each group to help facilitate the time-space-movement logistics of the testing program.

General teacher procedures

The use of smaller groups does not mean that these groups cannot be reorganized for different test activities. Some activities can involve larger groups, for example the endurance runs as contrasted with pull-ups. Therefore, as appropriate to the test at hand, multiples of a basic group can be incorporated to expedite the testing. For the sake of the reliability and the validity of the testing program, a carefully planned and conducted testing process is essential.

Become familiar with the details and objectives of each test event. Explain to the class the purpose of the test, and instruct the class in the correct procedures for each test event. Provide the opportunity for each student to perform the test correctly; ascertain that the testing stations are prepared, and that the necessary supplies and equipment are available.

Important points to remember

Observation of a student's performance in any physical activity is the first step in identifying physically underdeveloped pupils. In addition to observation of a student's performance, school personnel should use the following procedures:

Test Results Utilization

Identifying physically underdeveloped and obese students

- Obtain pertinent information from the student's physical examination.

- Review the student's growth pattern based on approved developmental criteria such as skin fold measurements. Performance on fitness tests is inversely related to obesity.

- Appraise the student's body balance and movement to determine whether the student has postural deviations that may restrict the student's achieving best performance.

Determine the student's physical fitness level on each selected test item. The student's performance at a given age may be appraised by interpreting the results as percentile scores. If the student's score is at or below the 25th percentile, it may indicate a physical fitness deficiency. Additional information which may explain poor performance should be obtained from the nurse or counselor. This information should include records of conditions, such as illnesses, accidents, poor eating habits, irregular growth, emotional problems, and physical handicaps.

Posture Check Report

Name _____ Grade _____ School _____

Date _____ Check made by _____

SIDE VIEW
Head
  Erect, chin in _____ Somewhat forward _____ Markedly forward _____
Upper Back
  Shoulders back _____ Slightly rounded _____ Rounded _____
Lower Back
  Slight natural curve _____ Moderately curved _____ Hollowed _____
Abdomen
  Flat _____ Slightly protruded_____ Protruded _____
Knees
  Relaxed _____ Slightly back _____ Hyperextended _____
Feet
  Pointed ahead _____ Pointed out somewhat _____ Pointed out _____

FRONT AND BACK VIEW
Shoulders
  Level _____ Slightly uneven _____ Considerably uneven _____
Hips
  Level _____ Slightly uneven _____ Considerably uneven _____
Backs of Ankles and Feet
  Heels and ankles
  straight _____ Turned out somewhat_____ Pronated _____

REMARKS

Class Posture Check

Class _____ School _____

Date _____ Teacher _____

Code
			Side View						Front and Back View			Remarks

Meets good postural standards 1
Slight but definite deviation 2
Marked deviation 3

Columns: Head and Neck, Upper Back, Lower Back, Abdomen, Knees, Feet, Level of Shoulders, Level of Hips, Feet and Ankles

Name
1.
2.
3.

When the majority of a class or school perform at or below the 50th percentile in one or more of the physical test events, the program should be critically examined, and activities in the program that contribute to the improvement of physical fitness should be increased. If overall results of the class show poor performance in the area of strength, the offerings in stunts, tumbling, self-testing activities, and activities on apparatus should be increased. If overall results of the class show poor performance in cardiorespiratory endurance, activities that require an increased length of time and distance in running, walking, and moving should be stressed. Such activities include relay races, soccer, speed-a-way, continuous rhythmical activities, and rope jumping.

When the majority of pupils in a class or school perform at or above the 75th percentile in one or two of the physical test events, the program of activities should be examined for a balance of all instructional units. Care must be taken to provide activities which will maintain the high level of performance. Care also should be taken to increase activities which will improve performance in areas of low achievement. Often entirely new units of instruction need to be introduced to meet the needs of certain pupils.

Planning the physical fitness program to meet class needs

Instruction is adapted to meet the individual needs of students by selecting specific activities which assist in the strengthening of weaknesses identified by the physical fitness test.

The teacher may find it necessary to provide an individualized program with a student at school and at home, with a small group or squad who have comparable deficiencies, or with the entire class. Management objective 5.2 details various computer programs and how each can be utilized to assist instruction by providing prescriptive developmental activities based on pretest information. Even if computer assisted instruction is not available, teachers should still attempt to individualize instruction for each student. One method is for the teacher to develop a physical fitness profile card on which physical fitness test scores, percentile rankings, and suggested developmental activities are recorded.

As students are tested, the raw scores should be compared to local, regional, state, or national norms and converted to percentile rankings. Percentile rankings represent the percentage of students of similar age and sex who scored at or below the provided test score. The higher percentage ranking represent higher levels of physical fitness.

Developmental activities prescribed should be designed to help each student develop higher levels of physical fitness. These prescriptions should tell students what specific activity or types of activities are needed to improve the physical fitness level in each component measured, how vigorously they need to do them, and for how long.

Individualizing physical fitness instruction to meet students needs

Sample Student Physical Fitness Profile Card

Name _____ Period/Room_____ Teacher_____

Date of Pretest _____   Date of Posttest _____

Age_____ Height_____ Weight_____   Age_____ Height_____ Weight_____

	Score	% Rank		Score	% Rank
One mile run	_____	_____	One mile run	_____	_____
Pull-up	_____	_____	Pull-up	_____	_____
Sit-up	_____	_____	Sit-up	_____	_____
Sit and reach	_____	_____	Sit and reach	_____	_____
Skin fold	_____	_____	Skin fold	_____	_____

DEVELOPMENTAL ACTIVITIES

Cardiorespiratory Endurance   Flexibility

_____   _____

_____   _____

_____   _____

Muscular Strength and Endurance   Body Composition

_____   _____

_____   _____

_____   _____

A list of activities which can be used to meet specific physical development needs can be found under Management Objective 5.6. The activities are grouped according to the primary components of physical fitness that are tested.

References

Dauer, V. and Pangrazi, R. 1983. *Dynamic Physical Education for Elementary School Children.* Minneapolis, MN: Burgess Publishing Company.

The Physical Performance Test for California. 1982. Sacramento: California State Department of Education.

Youth Physical Fitness. 1983. Washington, D.C.: President's Council on Physical Fitness and Sports.

Provide Professional Support to Staff on the Principles of Exercise and Instructional Approaches

Management Planning Steps:

Step One   Consult with staff and conduct inservice programs on the principles of exercise.

Step Two   Consult with staff and conduct inservice programs on the variety of instructional approaches that are available for teaching physical fitness.

Management Objective 5.4

Sample Principles of Exercise and Instructional Approaches

Principles of Exercise

Exercise tolerance—Factors such as fitness level, health, age, and developmental level of individual participants must be considered.

Warm-up—The body should be properly prepared just before a vigorous exercise session.

Cool down—The body should slow down gradually from a session of vigorous exercise.

Overload—An exercise session must be conducted at a level vigorous enough or intense enough to cause change.

Progression—The intensity, frequency, and/or duration of each exercise session must be increased over a period of weeks and months to continue to show improvements.

Specificity—The type of exercise engaged in and the particular body parts involved must be selected to meet the needs of the specific component of physical fitness to be developed.

Regularity—Exercise sessions must be conducted at regular intervals daily, weekly, and throughout the entire year to maintain or advance value gained from any physical fitness program.

Nutrition—The body requires appropriate quantity and quality of foods and a balance of caloric intake with exercise.

Sleep and rest— The body requires appropriate quantities of sleep and rest at regular intervals.

Harmful substances—Substances such as tobacco, alcohol, and drugs will decrease the body's capacity to perform at normal functioning and physical activities.

Recovery—The body requires an interval of time and periods of rest and sleep to recover from a vigorous exercise session. The amount of time needed for recovery is less for the physically fit person.

Summary of application of selected principles to physical fitness components

	Cardiorespiratory Endurance	Muscular Strength	Muscular Endurance	Flexibility
SPECIFICITY Exercise in a way to influence a particular component.	-Raise the pulse rate. -Best accomplished through continuous rhythmic activities such as walking, jogging, cycling, swimming, skating, and rowing. Sports such as soccer, basketball, racquetball may help.	-Make particular muscular groups exercise against heavy resistance.	-Make particular muscular groups do repetitions of exercise which requires strength.	-Move joints through full range of motion by stretching. -Use slow, static stretches, not quick movements.
OVERLOAD An exercise period conducted at a level vigorous enough by intensity and/or duration to get a training effect.	Intensity: -Raise the pulse rate to 60-90% of maximum pulse rate service. -Utilize 50-85% of VO² maximum. Duration: -Keep pulse rate up 15-60 minutes.	Intensity: -Use 70-80% of maximum resistance for each muscle group. Duration: -Do 4-6 repetitions in each set.	Intensity: -Use 40-60% of maximum resistance for each muscle group. Duration: -Do 8-15 repetitions.	Intensity: -Take each joint to maximum range of motion. Duration: -Go into each stretch slowly and hold 12-15 seconds. Repeat three times.
REGULARITY Exercise at regular intervals, each week, throughout the year.	Frequency: -Minimum of three days a week year round. Four to six days significantly better.	Frequency: -Minimum of two days a week year round.	Frequency: -Minimum of two days a week year round.	Frequency: -Daily, whether doing other exercise or not. Include as part of warm-up before vigorous activity. Repeat after activity for muscles used in that activity.
PROGRESSION Increases in the intensity, frequency, and/or duration over a period of time (weeks and month).	Intensity: -Go faster. Duration: -Go longer. Frequency: -Do the activity more times per week and/or per day. -Use combinations of intensity, duration, and frequency increases.	Intensity: -Use more resistance. Duration: -Do more sets. -Do the activity more times per week and/or per day. -Use combinations of intensity, duration, and frequency increases.	Intensity: -Use more resistance. Duration: -Do more sets. Frequency: -Do the activity more times per week and/or per day. -Use combinations of intensity, duration, and frequency increases.	Intensity: -Move joint to greater range. Duration: -Hold the stretch longer. Frequency: -Do the stretches more times a day. -Use combinations of intensity, duration, and frequency increase.

Instructional approaches

Program administrators have the responsibility to conduct staff development activities that will expand the traditional command style of teaching to include a variety of instructional approaches which enhance individual achievement. Program administrators also assume the responsibility to supervise the instructional program to ensure the implementation of effective teaching styles.

Lecture— TEACHER verbally presents the material.

LEARNERS record the material.

Drill— TEACHER provides a skill analysis and demonstration.

LEARNERS practice the skill to increase performance.

Socratic approach— TEACHER repeatedly poses questions.

LEARNERS search for answers.

Mastery learning— TEACHER designs specific objectives for more than one mastery level and provides for different rates of learning and immediate feedback.

LEARNERS are assured mastery of a specific level, before proceeding to the next level and work at their individual rates of speed.

Compentency-based learning—

TEACHER designs objectives that learners must achieve before advancing.

LEARNERS know exactly what they must achieve before advancing, eliminating performance gaps.

Individualized instruction—

TEACHER adapts the program to the special needs of individual learners through diagnosis and prescription

LEARNERS needs are met on an individual basis and they progress, uninterrupted, at their own rate of speed.

Programmed instruction—

TEACHER divides subject matter into small steps with each step building on the one preceeding it.

LEARNERS actively respond to one task at a time and receive immediate feedback.

Systems approach—

TEACHER move learners step-by-step through a systematic model that identifies all parts of the instructional process.

LEARNERS proceed step-by-step through the process.

Information processing—

TEACHER facilitates the processing of information.

LEARNERS process and retrieve information accurately and creatively, and pursue subject matter deeply.

Peer teaching—

TEACHER transfers teaching responsibilities to the learners and increases peer interaction.

LEARNERS assume responsibility for helping each other learn a skill.

Role playing—

TEACHER stages real-life situations and problems.

LEARNERS solve problems by acting out roles through improvisation.

Team teaching—

TEACHER shares teaching responsibilities with professional peer(s).

LEARNERS are exposed to more than one point of view during instruction.

Interdisciplinary approach—

TEACHER coordinates the physical education program with other subject areas.

LEARNERS integrate concepts which are central to physical fitness and nutrition with other disciplines.

Contract learning—   TEACHER assists learners in designing individual contracts.

LEARNERS learn to educate themselves in or out of the classroom.

References

Hayes, A. *Fit to be You.* Burbank, CA: Walt Disney Educational Media Company.

Personalized Learning in Physical Education. 1976. Reston, VA: American Alliance for Health, Physical Education, Recreation, and Dance.

Management Objective 5.5

> ## Provide Professional Support to Staff on the Importance of Understanding the Considerations Which Cause Physical Fitness Activities to be Safe and Provide Maximum Benefit
>
> ### Management Planning Steps:
>
> Step One   Consult with staff and conduct staff development on safety and health considerations.
>
> Step Two   Consult with staff and conduct staff development on environmental considerations.
>
> Step Three   Consult with staff and conduct staff development on warming up and stretching considerations.
>
> Step Four   Consult with staff and conduct staff development on cardiorespiratory endurance considerations.
>
> Step Five   Consult with staff and conduct staff development on muscular strength and endurance considerations.

Sample Program Considerations

Safety and Health Considerations

It is vital that teachers know as much as possible about their students' individual fitness levels and health or medical conditions which will have a bearing on participation in physical activity. Information can be accumulated to serve this purpose if the following procedures are followed:

1. Encourage continued supervision of pupils by a family physician or medical advisor and dentist, including periodic examinations and correction of remediable defects.

2. Develop a system whereby appropriate health information from the physician and family is given to the school nurse. Include the

necessary sharing of information with physical education teachers by the nurse.

3. Conduct appropriate developmental activities before students participate in vigorous activities.

4. Teach students the underlying principles for the fitness activities in which they are participating.

5. See that students are appropriately dressed before they are given the opportunity to participate.

6. Enforce rules of safety and discipline around equipment and during activity.

7. Remove jewelry during activity.

8. Conduct periodic checks on equipment to be sure it is operating properly.

9. Take appropriate safety measures such as the use of mats, off-limit areas, traffic patterns, and safe spaces between pieces of equipment.

Environmental Considerations

It is important that physical education teachers evaluate the environmental conditions in which students are exercising and make appropriate adjustments in the program when conditions call for it. Explanations of the reasons for these adjustments must be made to the student. This is, of course, a most "teachable moment" and one which might also be capitalized on by the science department.

Exercising in the Heat

The heat built up in the body during vigorous exercise is not harmful if the body has been conditioned to handle the heat and if it has a chance to get rid of this heat on a regular basis during and after the exercise. Perfectly normal body temperatures during vigorous exercise can range from 100° to 104° F. The ability of the body to get rid of this heat depends on its being conditioned through a regular, vigorous physical fitness program.

The temperature of the air is a big factor in the ability of the exercising body to rid itself of heat. So-called neutral air temperatures of 70°-80°F. cause significant body adjustments and students exercising vigorously in higher temperatures must be watched closely. The body gives off heat primarily through the cooling effect of evaporation of sweat from the skin. This occurs more readily if the air is dry rather than humid, if there is air movement, if the exercise is done in the shade rather than in direct sunlight, and if large areas of the skin are exposed to permit evaporation. Students should be taught to exercise in as little clothing as possible and still maintain appropriate decency.

Dehydration, loss of body fluid primarily through sweating, can be combated only by drinking water. Commercial drinks with a variety of additives are not needed by students in the ordinary physical fitness or sports activity in school. Excessive loss of salt in sweat can be replaced by adding salt to food at mealtime. This is rarely needed because most meals already have more salt than the body requires and excessive sodium from salt can be a health problem. Salt tablets should *not* be used. It is essential that students be encouraged to drink water according to their individual needs when they are exercising vigorously. This is particularly necessary when in a warm or hot environment. Vigorous exercise in rubberized suits or warm-up suits to promote sweating and weight loss should never be permitted. Students should be encouraged to drink about a glass of water 10-15 minutes before vigorous exercise, when considerable sweating is anticipated.

The more serious results of excessive body heat buildup are heat exhaustion and heat stroke. Even though their occurrences are rare, students should be taught the causes, symptoms, and emergency care procedures for handling such incidents.

Acclimatization to exercising in the heat can be lost in just a few days. Adjustments should be made for a class that has been exercising vigorously inside and then goes out into hot, direct sunlight. Individual adjustments must also be made for students who have missed two or more days of class.

Exercising in the Cold

Students should be permitted to wear appropriate additional clothing during colder weather. Some students may need to wear more clothing than others to maintain body heat. Stockings, hats, gloves, and/or warm-up suits should be permitted to encourage exercising in cold weather. As the individual warms up, extra clothing should be removed.

Temperature alone does not tell the amount of stress felt in the cold. The higher the humidity and/or the greater the wind speed, the greater the cold stress will be for the same thermometer reading. This is the chill factor.

Exercising in Air Pollution

Air pollution can be a problem in metropolitan areas. A school district should have a policy and implementation procedures covering physical activity during periods of an air pollution alert. This policy will usually be established jointly with the area air pollution control office. Teachers must know this district policy and procedures for compliance.

Carbon monoxide, which is a big part of air pollution, is attracted to the hemoglobin in the blood much more quickly than is oxygen. Therefore, the person breathing air with high concentrations of carbon monoxide will deliver less oxygen throughout the body and will be less able to exercise vigorously.

Warming Up and Stretching Considerations

The prevailing view of exercise scientists is that there is value in a warm-up period of low level activity just prior to more vigorous activity. The purpose of this is to prepare the joints, muscle tissue, and other connective tissues for activity and to gradually increase the activity of the heart and lungs. There are two kinds of activity during this low-level emphasis period before hard exercise: the traditional slow movement of all body parts generally called warm-ups, and flexibility exercises to increase the range of motion at particular joints.

The low level of physical activity by many persons and the large number of hours spent sitting in classes by students make it vital that a flexibility program be a part of the daily exercises in physical education. Flexibility exercises increase the range of motion needed to execute skills requiring this range more successfully. They are important in helping to reduce injuries to tissues around joints and to muscles during ensuing activities. Good flexibility in the low back associated with strong abdominal muscles will help reduce low back discomfort and can prevent chronic low back problems in adulthood.

Stretching exercises should be done every day. If a person is going to participate in vigorous activity, stretches should be done as part of the warm-up just before that activity. That warm-up should include other slow movements which relate to the particular activity (sport, game, dance, etc.)

The following points about stretching should be understood:

1. Slow stretching is best—no jerky or bouncing movements.

2. Muscles used during vigorous activity should also be stretched after the activity.

3. Each joint in the body must be stretched to develop or maintain flexibility in that joint.

4. A joint must be taken through increasingly larger ranges of motion over a period of weeks and months to increase flexibility in that joint.

5. Stretches should be done in all the directions that a joint moves.

6. Breathe with the stretch. Exhale slowly during the stretch and inhale while recovering position.

7. When doing any exercise that involves bending the trunk forward, exhale the breath while bending the chest toward the waist, and inhale when extending the trunk. This will minimize the internal pressure in the thoracic and abdominal areas.

8. Every person needs to do stretching exercises to develop or maintain flexibility.

9. Good flexibility will improve the use of skills in work or games and will help reduce fatigue.

10. Stretching exercises can be done during the day to relieve tension.

11. Good flexibility will help prevent injury and accidents.

Cardiorespiratory Endurance Considerations

The physical education activity schedule should include activities which develop and maintain cardiorespiratory endurance. Some can be attained through sports, games, and dance, but it is necessary to schedule long, slow jogging, running, swimming, and other similar activities to obtain adequate emphasis on this essential physical fitness component. Schedule more jogging/running when classes are in units like tumbling, volleyball, and softball, and less when they are in units like soccer and basketball. Make sure the same students are not always playing positions in games which are inactive (i.e., goalie).

Game rules can be modified to provide more activity. Examples: six players on a soccer team instead of eleven; football where forward or backward passes are permitted anywhere on the field and ball is alive until pass is incomplete or player is stopped according to regular rules.

Modifications for handicapped students can be made in the following ways so they can participate with other students:

a. Permit visually handicapped students to jog with a sighted student who is wearing a bell on a belt;

b. Permit handicapped to walk while others jog;

c. Use stationary bicycles;

d. Use rowing machines;

e. Use pool activities for those who can move in the water but not jog on a surface;

f. Provide arm cycle machines for students who cannot jog or cycle because of body, leg, or foot conditions.

Moderate intensity activity over a longer period of minutes is generally better than high intensity activity for a shorter period of minutes. A table to show the frequency, intensity, and time of exercise periods of cardiorespiratory endurance is as follows:

Fit Table

Frequency:	3 to 5 days per week
Intensity:	60% to 80% of maximum heart rate (220-age)
Time:	7 to 15 minutes of continuous exercise

Sports and games can be used by an individual for this component of fitness if the exercise of that individual in the game meets the above mentioned frequency, intensity, and duration.

Careful observation of children's reaction to exercise is an important part of the screening procedure. As has been stated, a poor reaction to exercise usually indicates poor physical condition rather than an acute or chronic disorder. However, it is advisable to check all questionable cases. If a child reacts poorly to exercise, the parents should be notified. If there are health care professionals associated with the program, the child should be referred to them.

Cardiorespiratory endurance is best developed when the activity is continuous and includes proper warm up, exercise, and cool down periods. Each period should be done at different heart rates to ease the transition from rest to exercise (aerobic) to rest. To do this, students should be taught the proper way to determine and monitor their pulse rate.

During the warm up period the pulse rate should reach approximately 140 beats per minute. During the exercise (aerobic) period between 140 to 180 beats per minute (target heart rate range), and during the cool down period should drop below 140 and approach 100 beats per minute. Target heart rate range is between 70 and 85 percent of maximum heart rate. Maximum heart rate is equivalent to 220 minus age of individual.

Monitoring Your Heart Rate

10 second count	× 6 =	Heart Rate	
17		102	
18		108	
19		114	
20		120	
21		126	
22		132	Warm-up
23		138	and
24		144	Cool Down
25		150	
26		156	
27		162	Aerobic
28		168	
29		174	
30		180	
31		186	
32		192	
33		198	
34		204	

TARGET HEART-RATE RANGE

Age	Maximum Heart Rate (220 minus age)	Target Heart-Rate Range (70 to 85 percent of maximum heart rate)
6	214	150-181 (beats per minute)
7	213	150-182
8	212	148-180
9	211	147-179
10	210	146-178
11	209	146-176
12	208	146-176
13	207	145-176
14	206	144-175
15	205	144-174
16	204	143-173
17	203	142-172
18	202	141-172

Here are the danger signals to look for:

- Breathlessness that persists long after exercise
- Bluing of lips that is not due to cold or dampness
- Pale, clammy skin or cold sweating during or after exercise
- Unusual fatigue
- Persistent shakiness after exercise
- Muscle twitching

There are other trouble signs that the teacher or leader cannot observe but which may be reported by boys and girls. If any of the following symptoms are recurrent after exercise, notification of parents and medical referral are recommended:

- Headache
- Dizziness

Obese children can seldom perform physical activities on a level with leaner children. This is due to the greater metabolic cost of exercise. Obese children require a higher oxygen uptake capacity to perform a task. Unfortunately, their capacity is usually lower than that of normal weight children which means that they must operate at a higher percentage of their maximum capacity. This forces the obese child to operate at a higher percentage of their aerobic capacity and allows them less reserve capacity. This lack of reserve probably explains why they perceive aerobic tasks as demanding and unenjoyable. Teachers would do well to bear this in mind when they ask obese children to try and run as far and fast as normal weight children. The task is more demanding of the obese child.

Muscular Strength and Endurance Considerations

The physical education activity schedule should include activities which develop and maintain these components of physical fitness. They will not develop adequately in students unless specific plans are made to include appropriate activity. There is a large number of boys and girls who are exceptionally weak in arm and shoulder muscles, and they need extra work in this area.

The amount of time spent on strength will depend on the number of days physical education is scheduled in a student's program. If students are scheduled for physical education four or five days a week, a good plan would be to consider the points listed below. If they have fewer days, it is unfortunate for them, and appropriate modifications will be needed to get as much fitness emphasis as possible, while providing appropriate instruction in other areas of physical education.

Conduct the screening test for muscle strength and endurance for all students and consider a student grouping plan so the underdeveloped will have more opportunity to improve in these components.

Handicapped students can easily be mainstreamed with regular students for most muscle strength and endurance activities. Minor adjustments in specific exercises can be made in accordance with individual needs.

Schedule each regular class to muscle strength and endurance activities (sit-ups, push-ups, etc.) two or three days a week throughout the year.

Schedule each regular class to a weight training station two or three days a week for the first month of the fall and spring semesters, and one day a week the remainder of the year.

Schedule each regular class to work at the chinning bars, climbing ropes, climbing poles, or peg boards for a few minutes, two days a week on a regular basis. Some classes can be scheduled at the beginning of the period and some at the end of the period.

There are many sports activities which will contribute to muscle strength and endurance development. Activities such as tumbling apparatus and wrestling should be a regular part of the physical education program.

References

Pestolesi, B. *Fun to be Fit*. Burbank, CA: Walt Disney Educational Media Company.

Hayes, A. *Fit to be You*. Burbank, CA: Walt Disney Educational Media Company.

Hayes, A. *Fitness for Living*. Burbank, CA: Walt Disney Educational Media Company.

Fitness for Life. 1983. Glenview, Illinois: Scott Foresman and Company.

Fitness Illustrated. 1983. New York: Boys Clubs of America.

Management Objective 5.6

Provide Professional Support to Staff on Conducting a Developmental Physical Fitness Program that is Concerned With Each Student's Present Level of Measured Physical Fitness

Management Planning Steps:

Step One   Consult with staff and conduct staff development on sequential developmental activities which increase flexibility.

Step Two   Consult with staff and conduct staff development on sequential developmental activities which increase cardiorespiratory endurance.

Step Three   Consult with staff and conduct staff development on sequential developmental activities which increase muscular strength and endurance.

Step Four   Consult with staff and conduct staff development on sequential developmental activities which increase flexibility, endurance, and muscular strength and endurance.

Step Five   Consult with staff and conduct staff development on activities to achieve optimal levels of body composition.

Sample Developmental Physical Fitness Activities

The sample developmental physical fitness activities in most sections are listed in order of difficulty. Some activities are appropriate for all students at the elementary and secondary levels and other activities are specifically designed for either elementary or secondary. A wide variety of activities are presented in order to meet the broad range of interests and needs of all students. Teachers should be reminded of the principles of exercise, especially specificity, frequency, intensity, and time, and also the variety of instructional approaches developed in Management Objective 5.4.

Sequential Developmental Activities to Increase Flexibility (Elementary through Secondary)

Shoulder Circles

- Start in standing position with feet hip width apart.
- Bend trunk forward slightly; bend elbows about 90° and slowly move elbows in large circles so stretch is at shoulders; do 10-12 circles with each arm.
- Stay in same body position and do free-style swim strokes with arms; be sure movement is slow and from shoulders; do 10-12 "strokes" with each arm.
- Stand upright and do backstroke swim strokes with arms; be sure movement is slow and from shoulders; do 10-12 "strokes" with each arm.

Side Stretch

- Start in the standing position with feet about hip width apart; clasp hands together and turn palms away from body; straighten elbows and bring arms up so they are touching ears and hands are overhead with palms facing upward.
- Keep the legs and hips in position and slowly bend trunk directly to the left side; keep elbows straight and right arm against ear; reach as far as possible over top of head with right hand; hold for four to eight seconds.
- Repeat step above going to opposite side.
- Repeat to each side three to four times.

Neck stretch

- Start in standing position with left arm over top of head and left hand on right ear.
- Keep the body in position and slowly pull the head directly toward the left shoulder; hold for four to eight seconds.
- Repeat step above to opposite side.
- Repeat to each side three to four times.
- Roll head slowly in full circles getting maximum stretch on all sides of neck; repeat six to eight times.

Knee Raises

- Start in standing position or lying on back.
- Raise right knee toward chest; keep upper body upright; place hands around right knee; slowly pull the knee closer to the chest and toward the left shoulder; hold for four to eight seconds.
- Repeat step above to opposite side.
- Repeat to each side three to four times.

Quadraceps Stretch

- Start in standing position or lying on left side.
- Raise right leg bent at the knee toward the back; keep upper body upright; grasp right ankle with right hand; slowly pull leg back so the knee moves back away from the plane of the upright body; hold four to eight seconds.
- Repeat above to opposite side.
- Repeat to each side three to four times.

Heel Cord Stretches

- Start in upright position.
- Step forward with the right leg so feet are separated a distance equal to about one half the individual's height; keep toes on both feet pointed straight to the front; bend right knee and lean forward; rest hands on right knee; keep left knee straight and left foot flat on surface; slowly lean forward as far as possible without raising left heel from surface; hold four to eight seconds.
- Repeat step above to opposite side.
- Repeat to each side three to four times.
- Assure position described in step above but bend left knee slightly and lean forward as far as possible without raising left heel from surface; hold four to eight seconds.
- Repeat step above to opposite side.
- Repeat to each side three to four times.

Ankle Stretch

- Start in upright position.
- Step forward with the right leg so feet are separated a distance equal to about one half the individual's height; keep toes on both feet pointed straight to the front; bend right knee and lean forward; rest hands on right knee; keep left knee nearly straight; lift left foot and extend left ankle so top of toes are on surface; roll ankle slowly as far as possible to the outside and to the inside of the foot.
- Repeat step above to opposite side.
- Repeat to each side three to four times.

Hip Stretch

- Start in upright position.
- Step forward with left leg so left knee is at about 90° angle and lower left is perpendicular to surface; keep right knee nearly straight; lower hips slowly until hands touch floor on either side of left foot; continue to lower hips as far as possible; hold four to eight seconds.

- Repeat step above to opposite side.
- Repeat to each side three to four times.

Lateral Hip Stretch

- Start in upright position.
- Spread feet so they are separated well beyond shoulder width; bend left knee and move hips toward left side; place hands on left knee; keep right knee straight and right foot flat on surface; lower hips slowly as far as possible; hold four to eight seconds.
- Repeat step above to opposite side.
- Repeat to each side three to four times.

Back Stretch

- Start in upright position, feet spread comfortably.
- Bend knees slightly; exhale while slowly bending forward letting hands, arms, shoulders, and neck muscles relax as much as possible; lower shoulders forward and down until hands are at surface; hold three to four seconds.
- Repeat three to four times.

Sequential Developmental Activities to Increase Cardiorespiratory Endurance (Elementary through Secondary)

- The children form a large circle and are spaced about six feet apart. The basic movement is a walk around the circle, not necessarily in step. The teacher gives various commands designating the activity to be performed.
- Most of these are locomotor movements which the children do while moving in the circle. The teacher may, however, direct the circle to stop and do certain exercises. After the task has been done, the children continue the walk around the circle.

Astronaut Drills

- The following movements and tasks can be incorporated into the routine: various locomotor movements such as hopping, jumping, running, sliding, skipping, giant steps, high on toes, etc.; on all fours, moving in the line of direction forward, backward, and sideward, repeat backward and forward using crab position; stunt movements like the Seal Walk, Gorilla Walk, Bunny Jump, etc.; upper torso movements and exercises that can be done while walking such as arm circles, bending right and left, body twists, etc.; various exercises in place. Always include an abdominal development activity. Children who lag can move toward the inner part of the circle and allow more active children to pass them on the outside.

Basketball Slide Drill

- The children are scattered on the floor or playground with each assuming a guarding stance as in basketball. One foot is ahead of the other and the hands are out as if guarding. The movements forward and backward should be made with a shuffle step with the feet retaining their approximate position. Movement to the side should be a slide.
- The leader stands in front with a whistle. He points in a direction and immediately the players move that way (forward, backward, or to either side). When the whistle is blown again, all stop. Other signals, such as "Go" or "Stop" could be used in lieu of a whistle.

- Another method to move the children is to station a player in front of the groups with a basketball. He dribbles rapidly in any direction, and the players move in relative position with him.

Endurance Hops

- Hops on both feet—up to 200.
- Straddle hops, laterally—up to 200.
- Scissor hops, forward and backward—up to 200.
- Hops on right foot—up to 50.
- Hops on left foot—up to 50.
- Squat-jumps touching hands to floor and springing upward again and again as long as possible (record total number of hops).

Fast Stepping

- Each child does very fast stepping in place just as rapidly as he can. This is kept up for ten seconds and then there is a ten-second rest. The cycle is repeated. This is quite strenuous and the children should be checked carefully to determine dosage.

Follow the Leader

- Lead group through the following: run around gym, jump across each mat, jog around the horizontal bar and to the far end of the gym and jump (long) rope twice before returning to starting place.

Knee Raised Run

- Run in place by raising knees as high as possible on each step. The arms should be swinging vigorously in each step. The weight of the body should be carried on the toes. The duration of running should be gradually increased to three or four minutes.

Rope Jumping for Time

- The object is to turn the rope as fast as possible during the time limit.
- The number of successful jumps is counted.

Running in Place

- Run in place by lifting knees as high as waist on each step. Carry body weight on front foot and toes. Each arm should swing rhythmically at the side of the body. The exercise should be performed first for a half minute and the time of performance gradually increased until three or four minutes duration has been reached.

Stride Hop

- With hands on hips, hop to a front stride position with left leg forward and right leg backward. Hop reversing position of legs with right leg forward and left leg backward. Repeat.

Walk, Trot, Sprint

- Children are scattered around the circumference of the room, all facing counterclockwise. The signals are given with a whistle. On the first whistle, the children begin to walk around the room in good posture. The next whistle signals a change to a trotting run. On the next whistle, the children run as rapidly as they can. Another whistle signals for them to walk again. The cycle is repeated as many times as the instructor feels is necessary.

The following fitness activities are aerobic activities. The games and activities are done over a prolonged period of time and attempt to move children at about 60% of their maximum capacity. These type of activities need to be conducted with a minimum amount of players on a team in order to maximize participation and increase exercise heart rates.

M. M. I. Volleyball (appropriate for 4-6 graders)

Activity:	Volleyball
Object:	More movement in volleyball. To get everyone involved in the game volley.
Rules:	The ball must be hit 3 times on each side of the net prior to being returned to the opponents.
Exception of Rule:	The ball does not have to be hit 3 times on the side of the net when the ball is blocked at the net.
Variations:	It is sometimes helpful when introducing the unit of volleyball to allow the ball to bounce once on each side of the net. This variation takes the pressure off the players and allows them to work on good form and proper techniwues of the overhead shot, dig, and set to the front court.
Evaluation:	The game interest will be much higher for all students and not just the most physically endowed players on a team

Bottle Ball Fitness Game (appropriate for 4-6 graders)

Activity:	Bottle Ball
Object:	Sustained movement over a prolonged period of time.
Rules:	The game is scored and played similar to paddleball or volleyball. The major difference is that it can be played on a tennis or volleyball court. The tennis ball may be put into play any way possible. A paddleball racquet or bottle racquet is used in place of a tennis racquet.
Variations:	May be played with partners or singles or teams.
Evaluation:	The fun in most games comes from the amount of involvement from the players. If all students are involved, they are having fun.

B. B. V. Fitness Game (appropriate for 5-6 graders)

Activity:	Basketball, Baseball, Volleyball
Object:	The ball must be hit, thrown, or batted using the various skills of (1) basketball, (2) baseball, and (3) volleyball. Choose teams appropriate for your class. Designate a team out in field and one team up to bat. After the batter has thrown, hit, or batted the ball, he must run around the outside of the basketball court while the players out in the field retrieve and pass the ball to each basket, whereupon the person under the basket must shoot and make the basket. The number of baskets depend entirely on your class size and running distance.
Rules:	Three outs retire a side. Fielders must rotate each play.

The person up to bat handles his own ball.

One point is scored when a player beats the ball around the courts.

Outs: If the ball goes around to each basket and back to home plate; if the ball goes around to each basket and the runner is hit with the ball.

Variations:	The batter varies his hitting, throwing, or batting depending on the specific skill desired for basketball, baseball, or volleyball.
Load Placement:	Cardiovascular system; develops general as well as specific skills.

Activity:	Running	**Endurance Fitness Game (appropriate for 5-6 graders)**
Object:	Set up an obstacle course around a track or any running area around school.	
Rules:	To stay on the obstacle course from start to finish.	

Items to be placed on the obstacle course:
Hurdles
Tires (students must step in hole of tire)
Cans filled with sand and a stick with a flag on it
Water pit similar to one used in a steeple chase (sawdust, port-a-pit, or baled hay may be used instead)

Load Placement:	Cardiovascular system; increased agility

Activity:	Endurance Movements	**Endurance Circuit Stations (appropriate for 5-6 graders)**
Object:	Regulate body movements to music	
Rules:	Continuous movement	

Circuit training is a teaching technique which effectively utilizes time, equipment, and facilities in conditioning programs. This teaching method provides incentive and motivation for all-out effort. A circuit consists of a series of exercises or a specific workout at numbered stations arranged in a consecutive pattern, either indoors or outdoors, in such a way as to enable persons to move easily from one station to the next. A circuit can be devised without equipment or can utilize gymnasium or outdoor apparatus. The time required to complete the activity at each station should be approximately the same to avoid congestion. The circuit's degree of difficulty can be increased or decreased to fit the needs of individuals or groups. The circuit can include stations for rope skipping, straddle hops, mountain climbs, ball bouncing, stride hops, running in place, and endurance hops.

Another variation for endurance movements is to have students in one large circle going in one direction. The students regulate their body movements to music and move continuously throughout the time period. The change of command from running to hopping, side straddle hops, rope skipping, stride hops or walking comes from the instructor rather than predetermined circuits. The commands should allow vigorous movements in combination with slow or recovery movements.

Running Programs (appropriate for 5-6 graders)

- Run for Fun—Program A. Run and walk for 20 minutes as desired. Stress good interval running.
- Staircase—Program B. Run 1', 2', 3', 2', 1', total of 12 minutes running, with 1 minute walking between run intervals.
- Staircase—Program C. Run 1', 2', 3', 4', 3', 2' 1', total of 16 minutes running time with 1 minute walking between run intervals.
- 3, 8, 3—Program D. Run 1', 2', 3', 8', 3', 2', 1', total of 20 minutes running time with 1 minute walking between intervals, except after the 8 minute run where 1 additional minute is spent walking for a 2 minute post exercise recovery heart rate.
- 12 minutes—Program E. Warm up with alternate walk and run at intervals of 1 minute for a total of 6 minutes. Run 12 minutes continuously and check your results with Cooper's 12 minute run chart.

Fitness Clubs:

Rules:	Establish a certain level or a criteria for eligibility. Make eligibility comparable to school fitness tests or state physical performance test. Must be performed weekly.
Types of Clubs:	Joggers Club, Sit-up Club, Pull-up Club.
Motivation:	Encourage self-motivation so that students do not feel they are being compelled to join a club. Post the results and club members' names inside the classroom area so that it is visible to everyone. Allow students enough time to meet weekly. Ideal time would be during a recess period or 2 days of alternate free choice period for physical activity. Allow the students to jog in pairs or a group.
Results:	Students enjoy the values, benefits, and prestige of belonging to a club.

Suggested Easy Three Days a Week Sixteen Week Jog-Walk Schedule (Secondary Only)

Always do warm-up and stretching exercises before jogging and repeat stretching exercises after jogging (fewer repetitions needed). Let each student go at own pace.

Schedule One—jogging for time

Week One:	Jog 2 minutes; walk 1 minute (5 times)
Week Two:	Jog slow 2 minutes; walk 1 minute Jog 4 minutes; walk 2 minutes (2 times)
Week Three:	Jog slow 2 minutes; walk 1 minute (2 times) Jog 6 minutes; walk 2 minutes
Week Four:	Jog slow 2 minutes; walk 1 minute (2 times) Jog 8 minutes; walk 2 minutes
Week Five:	Jog slow 2 minutes; walk 1 minute Jog 10 minutes; walk 2 minutes
Week Six:	Same as week five
Week Seven:	Same as week five

Week Eight: Jog slow 2 minutes; walk 1 minute
                     Jog 12 minutes; walk 2 minutes

Week Nine: Same as week eight

Week Ten: Jog slow 2 minutes; walk 1 minute
                     Jog 14 minutes; walk 2 minutes

Week Eleven: Same as week ten

Week Twelve: Jog slow 2 minutes; walk 1 minute
                     Jog 16 minutes; walk 2 minutes

Week Thirteen: Same as week twelve

Week Fourteen: Jog slow 2 minutes; walk 1 minute
                     Jog 18 minutes; walk 2 minutes

Week Fifteen: Same as week fourteen

Week Sixteen: Jog slow 2 minutes; walk 1 minute
                     Jog 20 minutes; walk 2 minutes

Schedule Two—jogging for distance

Week One: Jog slow 220 yards; walk 110 yards (5 times)

Week Two: Jog slow 220 yards; walk 110 yards
                     Jog 440 yards; walk 220 yards (2 times)

Week Three: Jog slow 229 yards; walk 110 yards (2 times)
                     Jog 880 yards; walk 220 yards

Week Four: Jog slow 220 yards; walk 110 yards (2 times)
                     Jog 1320 yards; walk 220 yards

Week Five: Jog slow 220 yards; walk 110 yards
                     Jog 1 mile; walk 2 minutes

Week Six: Same as week five

Week Seven: Same as week five

Week Eight: Jog slow 220 yards; walk 110 yards
                     Jog 1 mile, 440 yards; walk 220 yards

Week Nine: Same as week eight

Week Ten: Jog slow 220 yards; walk 110 yards
                     Jog 1 miles, 880 yards; walk 220 yards

Week Eleven: Same as week ten

Week Twelve: Jog slow 220 yards; walk 110 yards
                     Jog 1 mile, 1320 yards; walk 220 yards

Week Thirteen: Same as week twelve

Week Fourteen: Same as week twelve

Week Fifteen: Jog slow 220 yards; walk 110 yards
                     Jog 2 miles; walk 220 yards

Week Sixteen: Same as week fifteen

Sequential Developmental Activities to Increase Muscular Strength and Endurance

Specific for arms and shoulders (elementary and secondary)

Horizontal Bar Activities

- Hang on bar with back of hands toward face and body hanging with no support for a count of one and drop to an easy landing by bending ankles, knees, and hips.

- Hang on a bar with back of hands toward face and with body extended for increasingly longer counts (10 to 20); rest and relax between attempts.

- Hang on a bar with back of hands toward face and with knees brought up to chest and lowered to position.

- Hang with arms bent and with back of hands toward face; hold chin at bar level until arms tire and then lower body.

- Perform a sloth hang, also called ankle pull-up, by grabbing one end of the horizontal bar with both hands and swinging the body up and cross the legs over the other end of the bar. While hanging with straight legs along bar, pull chin up to bar; lower and repeat alternating sides of head to bar. Lower legs first when dismounting and do so before tiring.

- Perform at least two "chins" by pulling up with back of hands toward face.

- Perform a pull-up with the elbows slightly bent.

Mat Activities

- Walk on all fours the length of the mat.

- Run on all fours the length of the mat.

- Perform a seal walk around mat; drag legs along the floor as the arms and hands move the body.

- Perform a partner pull-up. One person stands astride a person who is lying on his back with his head and shoulders between the legs of the standing partner. Person on the floor raises arms and interlocks hands and wrists with the partner above. Partner lying on the floor then pulls up until his chest touches the clasped hands or wrists while his body is kept in a straight line with the weight on his heels.

- Perform a tip up or frog stand. Squat so that hands are flat on the floor, somewhat turned in, elbows inside thighs and pressed hard against knees, feet close to hands. Lean forward slowly and transfer the weight of body onto arms and hands at the same time lift toes from the floor. Hold this position for from 5 to 20 counts. Head should be held up to get good balance. Increase time in which position can be held.

- Perform a hand stand with support for feet. Performer stands facing partner. Place hands on the floor about shoulder width apart. Arms and legs should be fully extended, head thrown well up. Try to throw the feet so that they are caught by partner. Position is held by pointing toes as feet balance over raised head. The hand stand may be taught from a position of both hands and one foot on the floor. The free leg then, by a swing, pulls both legs up into the air. Many children can do a hand stand easily from a standing position.

Push-up Activities

- Wall push-up—start with feet 12" from wall, leaning against wall with hands in push-up position. Lower chest to wall, raise to starting position. Increase progressively to 36" from wall.
- Body raise—start in prone position, elbows even with ears, forearms on floor. Raise body, then lower to starting position.
- Back push-up—start in a back leaning rest position. Keeping body straight, lower, touching seat to ground.
- Knee push-up.
- Bench press progressively elevated.
- Push-up.
- Seal crawl.
- Push-up with feet progressively elevated.
- Bar dips—start in arm rest position, arms fully extended on ends of parallel bars. Lower body until angle of upper arm and forearm are less than a right angle. Push up to arm rest position.
- Wide-spread push-up—hands outside of shoulders.
- Hands together push-up.
- Back handed push-up—face hands with fingers pointing outward.
- Hand clap push-up—spring and clap chest at top of the rise.
- Push-up with weight on shoulders progressively increased.
- Hand stand with feet on wall, hands 18 inches out. Lower nose to floor and raise.
- Extension press-up.

Rope Climbing Activities

(Beginning—single rope)
- Lower body, hand under hand to lying position.
- Raise body, hand over hand to standing position.
- Rope chin-up.
- Climb with foot clamp.
- Climb using arms and legs—descend.
- Descend using stirrup.
- Make fast and rest.
- Climbing without use of legs.

(Intermediate—single rope)
- Climbing rope from a sitting position on the floor.
- Climb from mat in a full level position—descend same way.
- Climb in an inverted position—descend in the same position until head touches mat.
- Stand and seat mount (requires ability to tie a line hitch)
- Inverted hang.
- Rocking chair.

(Intermediate—double ropes 4' to 5' apart)
- Climb one rope, descend two ropes using legs.

• Climb two ropes 10', "skin-the-cat" three times, climb to top, descend. Special note: May use tuck to "skin-the-cat" but the half lever is more difficult. It is essential to have sufficient spotters and mats for all rope climbing activities at all skill levels. Students must be checked out at floor level before performing any rope activity.

Peg Board Activities (secondary only)

• Bent arm hang—Hang at lowest level on board, with two pegs, with elbows at 90 degrees.

• Horizontal travel—Place four pegs in bottom row; have student grasp two pegs on right or left side and move to opposite two pegs; pegs are not moved.

• Horizontal travel and back—Repeat number two above and return to starting position.

• Place peg—Have student hang with elbows at 90 degrees; remove peg with right hand and replace it in same hole; remove peg with left hand and replace in same hole.

• Repeat placing pegs—Repeat above a specified number of times.

• Horizontal peg change—Student grasps two pegs on lower left side and removing one peg at a time, moves with those pegs to lower right side.

• Horizontal peg change and back—Repeat above and return to starting position.

• Repeat horizontal peg change—Repeat number six a specified number of times.

• Climb up one level—Climb with two pegs from lower left corner to second level left side and back down.

• Up and over—Climb with two pegs from lower left corner to second level, move to right side, and move back to first level.

• Climb up two levels—Climb with two pegs from lower left side to third level and back down.

• Climb up two levels and over—Climb with two pegs from lower left side to third level, move to right side and return to lower level.

• Climb up three levels—Climb with two pegs from lower left side to top level and back down.

• Climb up three levels and back down—Climb with two pegs from lower left side to top level, move to right side, and return to lower level.

Specific for Abdominal Area (elementary and secondary)

Bent Knee Sit-up

Raise upper trunk to sitting position touching elbows to knees, lower to starting position.

Controlled Head Stand

Place hands on head on the mat so that they mark the points of an equilateral triangle. Move feet slowly toward face and raise hips to a position over shoulders. Raise one leg after the other or both legs at the same time until hips and knees, ankles, and toes can be held straight in vertical position. Return to the surface by bending hips and lowering legs so that the body weight can be taken on feet. (When a student is learning to perform the controlled head stand, a spotter stands with the side of his foot placed against the head of the performer on the mat. The side of the spotter's body provides a surface against which the performer's body may rest momentarily if the performer loses his balance while executing the head stand.)

Start in a supine position, arms crossed on chest. Raise upper trunk to sitting position, lower to starting position.

Curl-up

Start with back leaning against wall or partner's leg in a 45 degree position. Raise upper trunk to sitting position, lower to starting position.

Half Sit-up

Number one or bottom man must have strong shoulder muscles. He lies on back with knees bent. Number two man stands between his knees and as close to the bent hips of number one as he can. Three spotters should be used while this stunt is being learned, one to stand at each side and one at the head of number one. Number two places hands either on the knees or thigh of number one, according to the length of his arms, as he leans forward to allow his shoulders to be caught by the hands of number one. The elbows of number two must not bend, and number one must be careful to get a comfortable grasp on number two man's shoulders. Number two, by swinging one leg upward, raises both legs over his head. If number two remembers to point his toes and keep his head raised, he will have a perfect balance on the hands and knees of number one.

Hand-Knee Shoulder Stand

Start in a supine position, hands at side, palms down. Curl head forward. Lower to starting position.

Head Curl-up

Use incline board permitting feet to be higher than head. Raise upper trunk to sitting position and lower to starting position.

Incline Board Sit-up

Face and grasp bar with back of hands toward face. Swing legs backward and forward, and on forward swing bend arms and kick with one leg to bring hips to rest on bar with feet together. Hold a front-support position.

Pull Over (Hips Swing-up)

Lie on back. Lead with feet and roll backwards until hips are above shoulders and legs are extended vertically as high as they can reach with toes pointed upward. Maintain inverted body balance by bracing hands against body at the waist or a little below and resting upper arms on the floor parallel with body. Weight of body is carried on shoulders, neck, and elbows. Hold this position for several seconds and then return to original position by bending knees to chest, removing hand support, and slowly rolling from rounded back to pelvis, finally allowing legs to rest in place. Repeat until able to perform with no hand support.

Shoulder Stand

Sitting Tucks	Start in back sitting rest with legs 12" off floor. Pull knees to chest, push legs back to starting position and do not let feet touch the floor.
Skin-the-Cat	Jump upward, grasp the bar with back of hands toward face, and let body hang straight. Pull with arms, and at the same time, bring both feet between arms and under the bar. Continue to turn body between arms as far as possible. Release bar and land lightly on feet.
Up and Reach	Lie on back with arms extended beyond head. In one continuous movement lift arms, reach forward, and sit up. At the same time pull knees close to chest inside outstretched arms. Return to the starting position and continue to sit up and lie down in a rhythmical movement.
V-sit	Lie on back with legs straight and arms out from shoulders. Come to a position where body is balanced on the buttocks with the trunk and legs making a "V." Arms, stretched out from the shoulders, are used to balance. Return slowly to position. Repeat several times and try to hold the "V" position for a longer period during each performance.

Specific for Legs (elementary and secondary)

Endurance Hops (continuously)	Hops on both feet—up to 200; straddle hops laterally—up to 200; scissor hops, forward and backward—up to 200; hops on right foot—up to 200; hops on right foot—up to 50; and hops on left foot—up to 50.
Leap Frog	Number one player bends forward by supporting his hands on knees and ducking his head. Number two jumps over number one by placing hands on number one's upper back and jumping. Repeat four times alternating jumper.
Leap Frog Relay	Perform leap frog as a relay with six pupils in each line and leaping for a distance of 50 feet.
Pike Jumping	From a standing position, jump upward with both feet, keeping knees straight. Swing legs forward and touch toes with hands at top of jump. Repeat jump each five seconds for a specified time.
Stunts on Mat	Ankle pull—partners take a position on their hands and knees beside each other but facing in opposite direction. Each person holds his partner's nearest ankle with his hand and tries to crawl forward dragging the partner along. The person reaching the opposite side of the mat first is the winner. (Pupils should be matched according to size.)
Jumping the Square	Have the student sit erect, knees bent, heels on floor, with hands grasping toes. On command, have the student: straighten legs while maintaining hold on toes; return to the starting position; repeat the exercise. Teaching hints: stress "pushing" action of legs and "pulling" action of hands.

Have the student stand erect. On command, have the student: rise up on his toes on the count of "1;" return to standing position on the count of "2;" repeat the task. Teaching hints: Have the student perform alternately on right and left foot; have the student feel the calf muscle and explain what happened; increase time duration for holding No. 1 position; place text under the toes and perform.

Leg Straightener

Have student stand erect with arms at sides. On command, have the student: swing arms backward while bending knees; jump for height and distance, stretching arms over head; throw body and arms forward as he lands: repeat. Teaching hints: have the child jump repeatedly across the gymnasium and keep a record of the total attempts; vary by excluding the use of the arms, discuss the difference in distance resulting from the elimination of arm usage; record each student's best distance in inches.

Jump and Stretch

Weight Training (secondary only)

A well-balanced set of stations could include the following exercises:

• Bench press

• Arm curls

• Knee extensions (quadrups exercise) or half-squats

• Knee flexions (hamstring exercise)

• Upright rowing

• Bent over rowing

• Lateral arm raise

• Pull down (latisimuss)

• Spend considerable time at the start to test and help each student know the amount of resistance to use for each exercise.

Points to remember

• Be sure proper warm-up and stretching is done before each day's weight exercises are started.

• The general rule of thumb for muscle strength development—high weight (80% of maximum or more) and low repetitions (3-5). For muscle endurance—use lower weight (40-60% maximum) and high repetitions (8-12); do 2 to 3 sets on each exercise.

• For secondary school aged students, because of the limited time available, it is probably best to do 10-15 repetitions all the time to avoid strain and safety problems and to work on a combination of strength and endurance.

• Teach students to use good body position while doing weight exercises.

• If using free weights, use spotters where needed.

• Do not use the standing military press or dead lifts for this age. They can easily cause low back strains.

• Organize well so students know the order of movement from station to station for different exercises.

• If there are insufficient weights to have stations for an entire class, include some stations with developmental exercises like push-ups or sit-ups, or cardiorespiratory endurance activity like rope skipping, running in place, or bench steps.

Line activities (K-3)

- Line jumping sideward (side to side).
- Line jumping forward and back (front to back).
- Line scissor jumping (lead foot changes).
- Line jumping half turns (feet straddle line).
- Line hopping (side to side).
- Line hopping forward and back (front to back).
- Side stepping (use two or three lines).
- Line push-ups (front leaning position).
- Line hand cross (front leaning position), left, right across and left, right back.
- Line shuttle run (use two lines).

Activities to Increase Cardiorespiratory Endurance, Flexibility, and Muscular Strength and Endurance (Secondary)

A great variety of specific exercises of a heart/lung endurance nature and muscle strength or muscle endurance nature can be combined for vigorous and interesting fitness activity. By using records or tapes which are currently popular with students in the school, a creative, enthusiastic teacher can keep students involved in some fun activity that can meet criteria required to build or maintain specific components of physical fitness. This section will include a variety of examples from which other ideas will come easily to teachers and students.

Continuous Rhythmical Exercises

The following routines can be conducted in a gymnasium or small outside area, or on a large field or track. When done in a small area single, double, or triple lines can be used. Be sure to reverse direction several times when using a small area. Be sure to do warm-up and stretching exercises before starting.

Circular Continuous Workout: 5-7 minutes

(For gymnasium or equivalent size area—no equipment needed)
- Slow jog (low gear) around available area—once if large area, twice if small area
- Trunk twisting on each side—5 repetitions on each side.
- Slow jog around area (low gear).
- Side straddle hops (10).
- Jog around area (middle gear).
- Walk around area, shake legs, swing arms, breathe deeply.
- Push-ups (10).
- Hop on one foot around area alternating feet and occasionally using both feet (broad jumping).
- Slow jog around area (low gear).
- Straddle jumps (5).
- Balance on hands (frog stand)—10 seconds.
- Four count burpees (5).

- Jog, one lap (middle gear).
- Walk ½ lap, shake legs, swing arms, breathe deeply.
- Walk ½ lap on balls of feet, shake hands over head, breathe deeply.
- Five fast laps around area (high gear). If outdoors this could be replaced with one long run.
- Walk two laps, shake arms over head, walk on toes, shake legs, breathe deeply.
- Repeat stretches briefly.

Medium Gear Routine

- Jog ¼ mile, slowly, breathe deeply.
- Walk 200 yards with arm exercises (pumping and breathing, windmill, twisting with fingers laced behind neck), overhead shaking, flick-kick and arm shaking, deep breathing and forced exhaling).
- Run ¾ speed, 100 yards.
- Jog ¼ mile, slowly, breathe deeply.
- Walk 220 yards with arm exercises.
- Run ¾ speed, 100 yards.
- Jog ¼ mile, slowly, breathe deeply.
- Bent knee sit-ups (15).
- Jog ½ mile, slowly, breathe deeply.
- Walk 220 yards with arm exercises.
- Push-ups—maximum.
- Run ¼ mile, ½ speed.
- Sitting leg thrusts (15).
- Walk 220 yards—flick-kick and arm shaking.
- Side leg raisers—15 each side.
- Endurance hops—hands on hips (25 left foot, 25 right foot, 100 bouncing, 100 straddle, 100 stride).
- Jog ¼ mile, slowly.
- Walk 100 yards.

Count Down

This is an individual conditioning activity done in a group. Each student performs the activities listed, in order. The activities consist mainly of a series of runs followed by calisthenics or self-testing activities.

Jog	*Exercises*

5 laps	Abdominal Strength
	    V-Sit Up—10 times
	    Banana rock and roll—3 times

4 laps	Arm Strength
	    Full length push-up—10 times
	    Floor windmill (2 dip series)—3 times
	    Floor windmill (2 dip series)—3 times

(Roll to support position on right side, repeat to left side. Do 2 more times, 2 dips)

3 laps   Thigh Strength
           Limbo-Stix Windmill—4 times
               (Position body as if going under limbo stix; arms alternate to back, try to touch floor with hands)
           Downhill ski series—3 times
               (Knees and ankles tight together, ski. 4 jumps moving diagonally forward to left, same to right, do same action skiing 2 each way; lastly 1 each way 4 times)

2 laps   Back Flexibility
           Bridge series—2 times
               (Bridge position 1 count, hold; bridge position 4 count, hold; bridge position 8 count, hold)
           Wall series—2 times
               (Perform slowly—stand, back to wall 2-3 feet away, bend backwards and walk down wall 4 counts, gentle bounce 4 counts. Slowly come to stand)

Concepts and Activities to Achieve Optimal Levels of Body Composition

Concept: Body composition is a major component of physical fitness.

Definition: Body composition—the relative percentages of fat and fat-free body mass.

Overweight—a person who weighs more than other people of similar age and size is overweight.

Obese—a person who has an excessive amount of body fat is obese.

Activities: Discuss with students the difference between overweight and obesity.

Discuss the negative effects of obesity on posture, lower back, feet, and appearance. Also, explain that the heart muscle must work harder in the obese person.

Explain to students that the average male has 10 to 15 percent body fat and that the average female has 15 to 20 percent body fat.

Notes: It is possible for a muscular person to be overweight according to standard height/weight tables and still have a relatively small percentage of body fat.

- Students should understand that fat teenagers are more likely than average teenagers to become fat adults.
- The longer a person is fat, the longer and more difficult it is to lose the weight.

Concept: Body composition is related to diet.

Activities: Have students record the following for one week: when they eat, what they eat, how much they eat, and how long it takes to eat.

Have students record their daily caloric intake. Students can establish a program of weight loss or weight gain from this information.

Have each student evaluate personal eating patterns. If changes in eating patterns should be made, students should explain what these are and why these are needed. What insights did the student gain into personal eating patterns? Does the student eat foods that contain the proper nutrients? Does the student always, even when full, clean up the plate? How many snack-type foods does the student consume each day?

Notes: Students should be advised to get a medical checkup before beginning a diet. The physical education teacher should cooperate with the health teacher to coordinate this activity with a unit on nutrition.

Concept: Exercise and diet are directly related to weight control.

Definition: Calorie-unit of energy used to explain the value of food: there are 3500 calories per pound of body fat.

Activities: Discuss with students that there are three ways to lose weight:
- Dieting—to lose a pound of fat, a student must consume 3500 calories less than normally consumed.
- Exercise—to lose a pound of fat, a student must use 3500 calories more than normally used
- dieting plus exercise—to lose a pound of fat, a student must consume less and exercise more to achieve a combined reduction of 3500 calories.

Students should understand that a combination of dieting and exercise is the best method to insure weight loss and to improve physical fitness.

Notes: For a student to gain one pound, it is necessary to consume 3500 calories more than normal. A combination of dieting and exercise helps to lose fat and also helps to prevent the loss of lean body tissue.

Concept: Activity selection and duration is directly related to controlling body fat.

Activity: Discuss with students the activities on the Activity Energy Expenditure Chart and the number of calories used for each activity.

Have students determine how many hours they would have to perform different activities to lose one pound of fat. For example, if a student rides a bicycle for a half-hour every other day instead of watching television, six pounds of fat will be lost in one year.

Have students establish an activity program to aid in controlling body fat. This can be easily coordinated with the previous exercise programs students established in past activities dealing with the other components of physical fitness.

Notes: Students should understand that to lose a pound of fat they cannot increase their food intake. Exercise will reduce body fat as long as food intake remains the same or is decreased. If students desire to maintain or gain weight, they should be encouraged to exercise to improve physical fitness and also to increase their food intake. Exercise will help to increase and tone lean body weight. The teacher can combine this activity with a nutrition unit.

Activity Energy Expenditure

To determine calories used per hour, select body weight and match it with activity (i.e., a 150 lb. person will burn 540 calories during an hour of soccer).

Sports Activities

Weight (lbs.)	100	110	120	130	140	150	160	170	180	190	200
ARCHERY	180	192	204	216	228	240	252	264	276	288	300
BADMINTON	255	272	289	306	323	340	357	374	391	408	425
BASEBALL	210	224	238	252	266	280	294	308	322	336	350
BASKETBALL (half court)	225	240	255	270	285	300	315	330	345	360	375
BICYCLING (5.5 mph)	157	168	178	189	199	210	220	231	242	252	263
BOWLING	202	216	229	242	256	270	284	297	311	324	338
DANCE (aerobic)	255	272	289	306	323	340	357	374	391	408	425
DANCE (disco)	315	336	357	378	399	420	441	462	483	504	525
FENCING	225	240	255	270	285	300	315	330	345	360	375
FOOTBALL	225	240	255	270	285	300	315	330	345	360	375
GOLF (walking)	187	199	212	225	237	250	263	275	288	300	313
GYMNASTICS	232	247	263	279	294	310	326	341	357	372	388
HILL CLIMBING	367	391	416	441	465	490	515	539	564	588	613
HORSEBACK RIDING	180	192	204	216	228	240	252	264	276	288	300
JOGGING (5.5 mph)	487	519	552	584	617	650	682	715	748	790	833
JUDO/KARATE	232	247	263	278	294	310	325	341	357	372	388
JUMPING ROPE	525	560	595	630	665	700	735	770	805	840	875
RACQUETBALL	450	480	510	540	570	600	630	660	690	720	750
RUNNING (10 mph)	675	720	765	810	855	900	945	990	1035	1080	1125
SCULL ROWING	630	672	714	756	798	840	882	924	966	1008	1050
SKATING (roller/ice)	262	279	297	314	332	350	367	385	403	420	438
SKIING (cross-country)	525	560	595	630	665	700	735	770	805	840	875
SKIING (downhill)	450	480	510	540	570	600	630	660	690	720	750
SOCCER	405	435	459	486	513	540	567	594	621	648	675
SOFTBALL	210	224	238	252	266	280	294	308	322	336	350

Continued

Sports Activities

Weight (lbs.)	100	110	120	130	140	150	160	170	180	190	200
SWIMMING (0.25 mph)	232	247	263	278	294	310	325	341	357	372	388
TENNIS	315	336	357	378	399	420	441	462	483	504	525
VOLLEYBALL	262	279	297	314	332	350	367	385	403	420	483
WALKING (2.5 mph)	157	168	178	189	199	210	220	231	242	252	263
WALKING (3.75 mph)	225	240	255	270	285	300	315	330	345	360	375
WATER SKIING	360	384	408	432	456	480	504	528	552	576	600

Other Activities

Weight (lbs.)	100	110	120	130	140	150	160	170	180	190	200
DITCH DIGGING	300	320	340	360	380	400	420	440	460	480	500
DRIVING A CAR	90	96	102	108	114	120	126	132	138	144	150
GARDENING	165	176	187	198	209	220	231	242	253	264	275
HOUSEWORK	135	144	153	162	171	180	189	198	207	216	225
LYING DOWN (sleep)	60	64	68	72	76	80	84	88	92	96	100
MOWING THE LAWN	195	208	221	234	247	260	273	286	299	312	325
SITTING	75	80	85	90	95	100	105	110	115	120	125
STANDING	105	112	119	126	133	140	147	154	161	168	175
WOOD CHOPPING	300	320	340	360	380	400	420	440	460	480	500

References

Hayes, A. *Fit to be You*. Burbank, CA: Walt Disney Educational Media Company.

Pestolesi, B. *Fun to be Fit*. Burbank, CA: Walt Disney Educational Media Company.

The Physically Underdeveloped Child.. Washington, D.C.: The Presidents Council on Physical Fitness and Sports.

Priest, L. 1981. *Teach for Fitness*. Washington, D.C.: ERIC Clearinghouse on Teacher Education.

**Management
Objective
5.7**

> **Establish an Incentive Program Which
> Motivates Students, Staff, and School
> to Continually Seek Higher Goals
> in Physical Fitness**
>
> **Management Planning Steps:**
>
> Step One   Develop a motivation program for students.
> Step Two   Develop an award program for students.
> Step Three Develop an award program for staff and schools.

Sample Incentive Program

**Motivation
Program**

The general principles used in student motivation for physical fitness are the same as those used by teachers to create a positive learning situation for any aspect of physical education. An all-inclusive treatment of the psychology of learning would be necessary to deal with this topic completely, but that is not the intention here. The information in this section deals with some specifics that have been utilized successfully with physical fitness activities.

Physical education teachers should themselves carry out a personal physical fitness program so that they set an example for students to follow.

It is possible for teachers to do warm-ups and stretching, developmental exercises, jogging, or whatever other specific fitness activities the class might do, and thereby demonstrate to students that they believe it is important. This participation with the class should not be overdone because the teacher would not be meeting other teaching responsibilities. A good plan might be to do all of the fitness exercise with one class a day. By selecting one during each day and a different one each day of the week, the teacher could cover all classes and assist in maintaining his/her own fitness.

Because physical education teachers usually have been vigorous, successful participants during their lives, they must practice particular patience and understanding with the variety of inactive, underdeveloped, unskilled students in their classes.

Teachers should provide individually planned fitness programs utilizing test results, health information, education strategies, and counseling techniques.

Teachers can set up competition between squads or teams in a class or between classes to see how far each group can run, the number of pull-ups, of sit-ups completed, etc., in a day, a week, a month, etc. Establish several measured cross-country type courses around the school grounds to provide variety in running. Establish school or club cards for 100-mile club, 500-mile club, etc.

Competition by mail with nearby or far-away schools or clubs is a good motivator. Keep recognition boards in the locker room or school lunch room with names/pictures of school fitness record-holders, Presidential Physical Fitness Award Winners, etc.

This award is for children and youth ages 10-17 who score at or above the 85th percentile on each of the test items on the AAHPERD Youth Fitness Test. It consists of an emblem and a certificate. Colorful stick-on decals are also available.

AAHPERD has an award program for students taking the AAHPERD Youth Fitness Test which include standard emblems for 50th percentile achievement for elementary, junior, and senior high school students and merit emblems for scoring at the 80th percentile on all test items.

A new award program for students taking the AAHPERD Health Related Physical Fitness Test is available for those scoring at the 50th to 84th percentile. Fitness Award Certificates, Gold Merit Seals, and emblems for elementary, junior, and senior high school students may be earned.

Current prices, qualifying scores, and ordering information for the above student awards are available from the American Alliance for Health, Physical Education, Recreation, and Dance (AAHPERD), 1900 Association Drive, Reston, Virginia 22091.

Establish local fitness awards for various activities, or events, such as Super-Star Competition, Fitness Trails, Rope Skipping, etc.

This program is designed to help motivate local students, ages 10-18, to achieve physical fitness and to honor those students who demonstrate a high level of physical performance. The program allows students to receive two awards—the President's Physical Fitness Award and the Standard Physical Fitness Award.

Any school or district in San Diego County may participate in the program. Students become eligible for both awards by performing at prescribed achievement levels in each of the six test events in cluded in *The Physical Performance Test for California.*

The awards program, is sponsored cooperatively by the Ninth District, Inc., California Congress of Parents, Teachers, and Students (SSPTS), CCAHPERD—San Diego Unit; the San Diego Unified School District; and the San Diego County Office of Education. County and local school districts cooperate in helping identify recipients of either or both awards. The award materials to be given to students can now be purchased locally, using nonschool funds, from the Ninth District, Inc. CCPTS.

This award is given each school year for the large, medium, and small schools in each state with the highest percentage of eligible students who qualify for the Presidential Physical Fitness Award. Winning schools receive a handsome plaque and each student who qualifies for the Presidential Physical Fitness Award receives a special emblem and certificate. It is the responsibility of the school to make application. Application forms are available from the following sources:

- PCPFS, Washington, DC 20201

- AAHPERD, 1900 Association Drive, Reston VA 22091

Program administrators should establish an awards system that gives recognition to instructors who have best achieved established criteria for a sound physical fitness program.

Student Awards

Presidential Physical Fitness Award

AAHPERD Youth Fitness Test Awards

AAHPERD Health Related Physical Fitness Test Awards

Local Awards

San Diego Physical Fitness Award Program

School and Staff Awards

State Champion Physical Fitness Award

Staff Awards

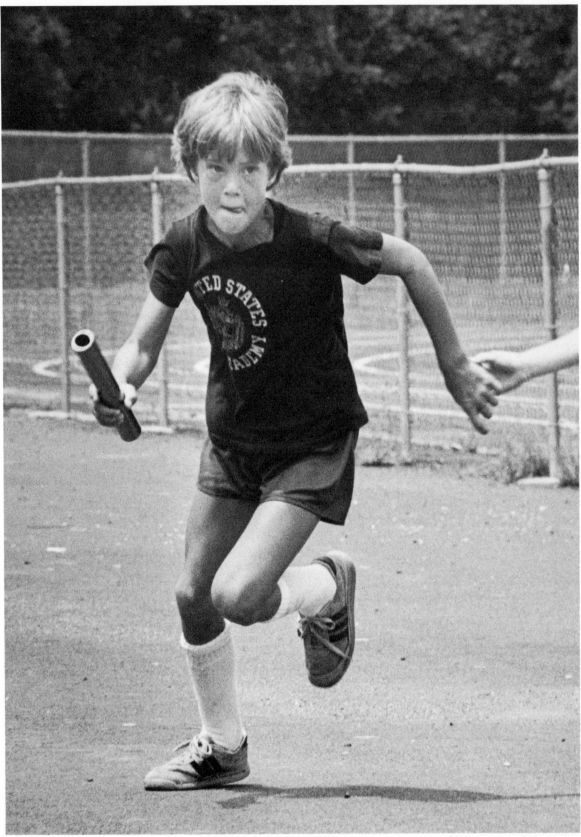

Photo courtesy Greg Merhar.

6.0

PUBLIC RELATIONS

Includes suggestions for developing a public relations plan, communication techniques to publicize the program, and plan for regular exhibitions and demonstrations.

**Management
Objectives**

**Management
Objective
6.1**

> ## To Build Community Support by Developing An Ongoing Public Relations Program for the Purpose of Creating Awareness of the Value of Physical Fitness
>
> **Management Planning Steps:**
>
> Step One   Develop a public relations plan for students, parents, administrators, school boards, and community.
>
> Step Two   Develop communication techniques to publicize the program.
>
> Step Three   Develop a plan for regular exhibitions and demonstrations.

Sample Community Support Program

Public Relations Plan

- Conduct a poll to identify community attitudes toward physical fitness.
- Develop a multimedia promotional program for physical fitness in your school and community.
- Contact service organizations, talk shows, and clubs in your community with offers to be placed on their programs.
- Send regular news releases about your physical fitness program to your local newspaper.
- Invite school board members and administrators to observe your instructional program. Discuss with them the objectives of your program.
- Make presentations at various educational and administrative professional conferences.
- Give recognition, in a public setting, to individuals from your school, community, and legislature who support physical fitness.

**Communication
Techniques**

The mass communications media—newspapers, radio, and TV—offer many opportunities for enhancing the physical fitness image and cultivating support. Again, programs which are achievement- or goal-oriented have a big advantage over recreational programs. The number and names of students winning Presidential Physical Fitness Awards, or a comparison of local fitness scores with state and national averages, are news in most communities. Reports on programs which serve the handicapped and retarded, or programs which teach useful skills such a swimming and drown-proofing, are also newsworthy.

It is usually helpful to assign responsibility for program publicity to a staff member with interest and aptitude in the activity. All releases should be coordinated with school and/or district public information officers, since they may have additional resources and contacts which will be useful.

Periodic reports to the principal, superintendent, and board of education are another means of interpreting the physical fitness program. Others include leaflets (explaining the scope and objectives of the program) which students take home to parents; photographic displays in window space provided by local merchants; interesting pictures and charts posted on school bulletin boards; display boards (in school gymnasiums or trophy cases) listing physical fitness record-holders; and color slides or movie film for use in presentations to PTA's, service clubs, fraternal organizations, etc.

An opportunity often overlooked by the physical educator is the local radio or TV "talk show." Such shows are an excellent forum for detailed discussions, and physical education has many friends in medicine—pediatricians, orthopedists, cardiologists, psychiatrists, etc.—who can contribute to interesting and informative presentations.

Exhibitions and Demonstrations

Exhibitions at school assemblies and at the intermissions of athletic events are perhaps the best means of reaching the public, administration, fellow faculty members, and students. Special "days" or "nights," which may be conducted by a single school or on a city-wide or district-wide basis, are effective for taking the message to the public. Each secondary school should conduct at least one demonstration annually, apart from the usual Back-to-School Night. Since experience indicates that such demonstrations attract approximately three adult spectators for each student participant, it is important to involve as many students as is practical.

Following are five examples of demonstrations whereby schools or districts can tell their stories effectively.

Sports-A-Rama (single high school)

Competing teams are formed by the four grades of the school. Seniors are indentified by their green trunks; Juniors, gold; Sophomores, blue; and Freshmen, red. Teams are judged according to precision and appearance in marching on and off the floor and during the warmup. First is awarded 50 points; second, 30 points; third, 20 points; and fourth, 10 points. Decoration of their assigned sections of the bleachers by classes is awarded: first, 100 points; second, 60 points; third, 40 points; fourth, 10 points. Cheering and enthusiasm of classes is awarded; first 100 points; second, 60 points; third, 40 points; fourth, 20 points.

Sports-A-Rama (1-hour, 45-minute program)

7:30-7:35	Grand March and Warmup	All classes
7:35-7:40	Sports-A-Rama Song	Song leaders
7:40-7:45	Volleyball (10 points)	Seniors vs. Juniors (6 men on a team)
7:45-7:48	Wheelbarrow Relay (10 points)	Sophomores vs. Juniors (8 men on a team)
7:48-7:51	Basketball Relay (10 points)	Seniors vs. Sophomores (8 men on a team)
7:51-7:54	Knee Basketball (10 points)	Juniors vs. Sophomores (3 men on a team)
7:54-7:57	Standing Jump Relay (10 points)	Freshmen vs. Sophomores (8 men on a team)

7:57-8:00	Tumbling RelaySeniors vs. Freshmen	
	(10 points) ....(8 men on a team)	
8:00-8:05	Tug of War....................................... All classes	
	Single Elimination ....(40 men on a team)	
	Freshmen vs. Juniors, Sophomores vs. Seniors	
8:05-8:08	Dizzy Izzy Relay ....Seniors vs. Sophomores	
	(10 points) ....(8 men on a team)	
8:08-8:11	Sack Race .... Freshmen vs. Juniors	
	(10 points) ....(8 men on a team)	
8:11-8:14	Crab Race .... Seniors vs. Freshmen	
	(10 points) ....(8 men on a team)	
8:14-8:19	Push Ball .... Juniors vs. Seniors	
	(10 points) ....(8 men on a team)	
8:19-8:22	Barrel Relay.................... Freshmen vs. Sophomores	
	(10 points) ....(8 men on a team)	
8:22-8:25	Stroke-the-Boat Race .... Juniors vs. Freshmen	
	(10 points) ....(8 men on a team)	
8:25-8:35	Pyramid Building................................All classes	
	Judged on organization, difficulty, achievement, and number of students used. 1st—100 points; 2nd—60 points; 3rd—40 points; Entry—20 points	
8:35-8:55	Individual Contests............................ All classes	
	1st—10 points; 2nd—6 points; 3rd—4 points; Entry—2 points	
8:35-8:55	Individual Contests............................ All classes	
	1st—10 points; 2nd—6 points; 3rd—4 points; Entry—2 points	
8:35-8:45	Group A .... Weight Lifting / Tire Wrestle / Bulldog Pull / Tumbling / Rope Climbing	
8:45-8:55	Group B ....Indian Wrestle / Free Throws / Bar Dips / Elbow Wrestle / Pullups	
8:55-9:10	Obstacle Race ....All classes	
	1st—40 points; 2nd—30 points; 3rd—20 points; Entry—10 points	
9:10-9:15	Presentation of Sports-A-Rama Trophy by Principal	

Warm up exercises ....Girls and boys
Folk Dances in Native Costumes .... Girls
Relays (Circular and Shuttle)............................. Boys
Tumbling and Gymnastics ....Girls and boys
Modern Dance .... Girls
Circuit Courses .... Boys
Agility Response Drills .... Boys

Prelude—High school band
Presentation of Colors—AFROTC
Introduction of dignitaries and members of district board of education
   by Coordinator of Physical Education
Introductory remarks by State Physical Education personnel
Description of demonstrations and narration during activities by
   District Consultant in Physical Education and State Physical
   Education Chief

Demonstrations (Elementary Schools):

Gymnastics (Primary)	Creative Rhythms
Ball Handling Skills	Circuit Training
Balance Beam	Movement Exploration
Vaulting Box	Gymnastics (Intermediate)
Grass Drills	Parachute Play
Astronaut Drills	Stretch Ropes
Physical Fitness Development	Special Education Techniques
German Free Movement	Folk and Square Dancing

Demonstrations (Secondary School Girls):
   Junior High—Free Exercise, Tumbling
   Junior High—Modern Gymnastics
   Junior High—Modern Dance, Aerial Tennis
   Junior High—Jump Rope
   High School—Gymnastics Apparatus, Circuit Training
   High School—Golf, Badminton

Demonstrations (Secondary School Boys):
   Junior High—Pre-Tennis
   Junior High—Rope Climbing, Tumbling
   Junior High—Wrestling, Handball
   Junior High—Physical Fitness Testing
   Junior High—Gymnastics Apparatus, Physical Fitness Conditioning
   High School—Weight Training, Archery

25 yard dash	Reach and jump	Pull-ups
Rope climb	Standing broad jump	

Each youngster is limited to one event. Three team events are run off
in heats of three teams each. In the shuttle relay, obstacle relay, and
tug-of-war, teams are composed of two boys and two girls. Each team
member, in succession, completes these activities in the obstacle relay:

   Run 25 yards
   Climb through an automobile tire
   Walk a balance beam
   Climb over a 5′ Swedish vaulting box

Hurdle a 2' crossbar
Climb a 15' rope
Reverse the entire course
The tug-of-war team is composed of three boys and three girls

**Sports-A-Rama
(all county schools 11-12)**

7:30-7:33	Sports-A-Rama Song			
7:33-7:45	Calisthenics			
7:43-7:46	Physical Performance Test			
7:46-8:00	Court	Game	Court	Game
	1	Netball	5	Deck tennis
	2	Semi-volleyball	6	Volleyball
	3	Volley tennis	7	Paddle tennis
	4	Pushball	8	Badminton

8:00-8:05   Body Mechanics (Posture)

8:05-8:10   Crossfire (dodgeball game)

8:10-8:15   Scrimmage (basketball leadup game)

8:15-8:18   Passball (football leadup game)

8:18-8:21   Pushball

8:21-8:35   Dance and Basic Rhythms
Primary (fundamentals and creative)
Intermediate (folk and contra)
Upper grades (social)

8:35-8:40   Rope climbing

8:40-8:50   Base Games (baseball leadup games)
Primary—Homeball
Intermediate—Kickball and teeball

8:50-8:56   The Dance
Intermediate (Interpretive)
High School (Modern)

8:56-9:05   "Rasslin" and Wrestling

9:05-9:30   Tumbling and Trampolining

References

Pestolesi, B. 1985. *Physical Education: A Lifetime Commitment.* (Slide/tape promotional packet). AAHPERD Southwest District.

Physical Education Framework for California Public Schools. 1985. Sacramento: California State Department of Education.

Seiter, M. and Goggin, M. 1983. *Shaping the Body Politic.* Reston, VA: American Alliance for Health, Physical Education, Recreation, and Dance.

Youth Physical Fitness. 1984. Washington, D.C.: President's Council on Physical Fitness and Sports.

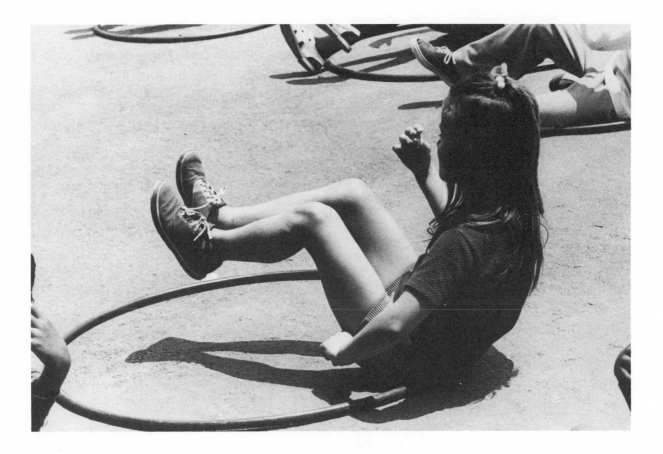

PROGRAM SUPERVISION AND EVALUATION

Includes a procedure for program supervision and program evaluation by listing various functions in supervising and evaluating each Management Objective.

Management Objectives

**Management
Objective
7.1**

**Supervise and Evaluate Operation of the
Children/Youth Physical Fitness
Program Management System**

Management Planning Steps:

Step One   Perform supervisory functions as necessary for
            successful system operation.

Step Two   Evaluate effectiveness level of each manage-
            ment objective of the program management
            system.

Sample Program Supervision
and Evaluation Functions

**Program
Supervisory
Functions**

It is the function of the program manager to supervise the sequential
management planning steps to ensure the completion of each management objective. A check list of supervisory functions is included to
meet this responsibility.

For successful supervision to take place, it is essential that the
program administrator is democratic, "people oriented," and able to
see situations as others do. The supervisor should be a model, a leader,
a teacher of teachers, and must exemplify all that is best in con-
temporary teaching by stimulating professional growth among the
teachers with whom they work.

**Program
Evaluation Criteria**

The program administrator must evaluate effectiveness of the
program management system. The system evaluation criteria that
follows measures the completion level of the various management
objectives. This evaluation process becomes a check list of objective
attainment and should assist the administrator in program management. A good evaluation process will provide essential information to
teachers, administrators, and community as to how the school or
district is progressing in implementation of a physical fitness program.

Check List of Supervisory Functions and Criteria for Evaluating Each Management Objective

Check (✔) functions and criteria as completed

Management Objective	Supervisory Functions	Evaluation Criteria
1.1 Determine the operational level for each management stage of your children/youth physical fitness system.	____ Conducted an assessment of your program utilizing the Program Management System Assessment instrument provided. ____ Set priorities and established strategies for program development or revision.	____ Operational level of your Program Management System has been determined, priorities set, and strategies for program development or revision established.
2.1 Enlist support and commitment for a children/youth physical fitness program.	____ Compiled a packet of support materials justifying the needs and purposes for a physical fitness program. ____ Enlisted commitment from the instructional staff to conduct a strong physical fitness program at all levels. ____ Obtained support from the local governing board, school administrators, and community for a continued program.	____ Support and commitment for a comprehensive school physical fitness program at all levels has been granted.
3.1 Develop a physical fitness program as a part of the total physical education curriculum.	____ Assisted writing committee in developing a philosophy statement. ____ Assisted writing committee in developing program goals. ____ Assisted writing committee in developing program concepts. ____ Assisted writing committee in developing student objectives. ____ Assisted writing committee in developing learning experiences for each grade level.	____ A physical fitness curriculum has been developed which includes a philosophy statement, program goals, concepts, student objectives, and learner experiences.
4.1 Determine the legal statutes which govern the physical fitness program as part of regular physical education instruction.	____ Determined the legal foundations for the program based on federal statutes. ____ Determined the legal foundations for the program based on state statutes.	____ Federal and state statutes that govern your physical fitness program have been identified and adopted.

Continued

Management Objective	Supervisory Functions	Evaluation Criteria
4.2 Develop an operational budget to support the physical fitness program.	_____ Determined the physical fitness budget expenditure classifications. _____ Determined the annual funding necessary for a minimal physical fitness program at each school. _____ Determined the annual funding necessary for an expanded physical fitness program at each school.	_____ A budget has been developed and approved which includes necessary resources to operate your physical fitness fitness program.
4.3 Staff the school or department with credentialed teachers qualified to teach the concepts and practices of physical fitness to all students as part of a regular measure-physical fitness education program.	_____ Specified strengths necessary related to biological, psychological, and sociological foundations. _____ Specified strengths necessary related to instruction. _____ Specified strengths necessary related to measurement and evaluation.	_____ Staff have been employed to teach physical fitness that possess strengths in biological, psychological, and sociological foundations instruction, ment and evaluation, and organization and administration.
4.4 Provide for facilities and equipment that will enhance the physical fitness component.	_____ Surveyed existing indoor and outdoor physical fitness facilities. _____ Surveyed existing indoor and outdoor physical fitness equipment. _____ Set priorities and strategies for acquisition of new physical fitness facilities and equipment.	_____ Adequate physical fitness facilities and equipment are provided.
4.5 Provide appropriate instructional materials and supplies for effective instruction.	_____ Surveyed available instructional materials, audio-visual aids, and program _____ Established priorities for purchase of instructional materials, audiovisual aids, and program supplies. _____ Arranged for program implementation of the materials and supplies.	_____ Appropriate instructional materials and supplies for effective physical fitness instruction are provided.

Management Objective	Supervisory Functions	Evaluation Criteria
5.1 Establish a physical fitness testing program that will assess the physical fitness level of all students.	_____ Determined if my state mandates a particular physical fitness test. _____ Selected a national physical fitness test or approved test items if state does not mandate one.	_____ A physical fitness testing program that assesses the level of all students is utilized.
5.2 Incorporate a computerized physical fitness program to facilitate instruction.	_____ Determined type of physical fitness computer assisted programs needed that are compatible with our test battery. _____ Recommended software for purchase which match program needs and computer hardware available.	_____ Appropriate computer software to facilitate physical fitness instruction is provided.
5.3 Provide professional support to staff on administration and utilization of test results.	_____ Consulted with staff and conducted staff development on appropriate physical fitness test administration. _____ Consulted with staff and conducted staff development on utilization of test results.	_____ Staff have been informed on physical fitness test administration and utilization of test results.
5.4 Provide professional support to staff on the principles of exercise and instructional approaches.	_____ Consulted with staff and conducted staff development on the principles of exercise. _____ Consulted with staff and conducted staff development on the variety of instructional approaches to physical fitness instruction.	_____ Staff have been informed on the principles of exercise and the various instructional approaches to teaching physical fitness.
5.5 Provide professional support to staff on the importance of understanding the considerations which cause physical fitness activities to be safe and provide maximum benefit.	_____ Consulted with staff and conducted staff development on safety and health considerations. _____ Consulted with staff and conducted staff development on environmental considerations. _____ Consulted with staff and conducted staff development on warming up and stretching considerations.	_____ Staff have been informed on the importance of understanding the considerations which cause physical fitness to be safe.

Continued

Management Objective	Supervisory Functions	Evaluation Criteria
	_____ Consulted with staff and conducted staff development on cardiorespiratory endurance considerations. _____ Consulted with staff and conducted staff development on muscular strength and endurance considerations.	
5.6 Provide professional support to staff on conducting a developmental physical fitness program that is concerned with each student's present level of measured physical fitness.	_____ Consulted with staff and conducted staff development on activities which measure flexibility. _____ Consulted with staff and conducted staff development on activities which measure cardiorespiratory endurance. _____ Consulted with staff and conducted staff development on activities which increase flexibility, endurance, and muscular strength and endurance. _____ Consulted with staff and conducted staff development on concepts and activities to achieve optimal body composition.	_____ Staff have been informed on how to conduct an individualized developmental physical fitness program.
5.7 Establish an incentive program which motivates students, staff, and school to continually seek higher goals.	_____ Developed a motivation program for students. _____ Developed an award program for staff and schools.	_____ An incentive program which motivates students, staff, and school to achieve higher goals in physical fitness is established.
6.1 Build community support by developing an ongoing public relations program for the purpose of creating awareness of the value of physical fitness	_____ Developed a public relations plan for students, parents, administrators, school boards, and community. _____ Developed communication techniques which publicize the physical fitness program. _____ Developed a plan to conduct regular exhibitions and demonstrations.	_____ A public relations program which keeps the community aware of the school physical fitness program is established.

Management Objective	Supervisory Functions	Evaluation Criteria
7.1 Supervise and evaluate operation of the children/youth physical fitness program management system.	_____ Performed supervisory functions as necessary for successful program management system operation. _____ Evaluated effectiveness level of each management objective of the program management system.	_____ The children/youth physical fitness program management system has been supervised and evaluated.

Completion of the supervisory check list for evaluating each objective of the physical fitness management system will provide information to the user as to the success level and completion of the various steps in achieving established program goals.

It is the responsibility of the program administrator to use this information as a guide or referral to the appropriate management stage or objective for completion. Effective use of this tool will provide a sequential pattern of referral that will result in a continuous evaluation of program development leading to the continued successful operation of the management system.